5/11

DISCARD

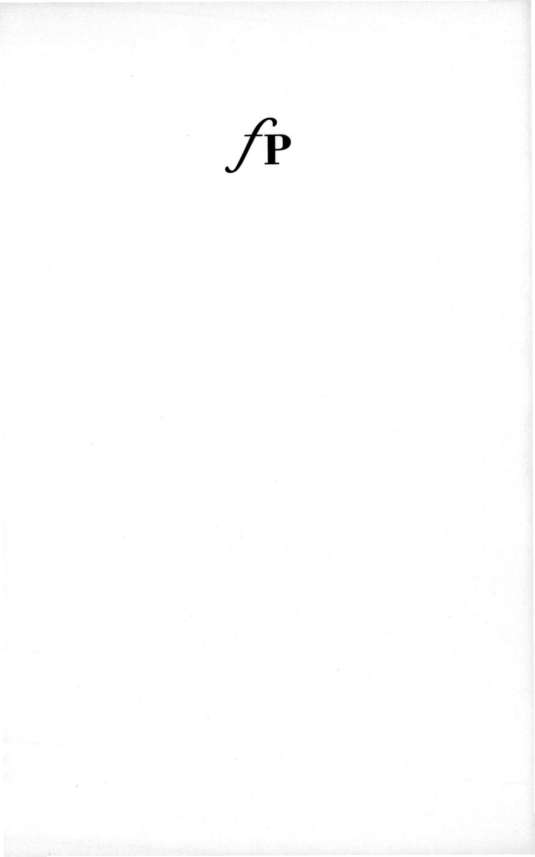

Alzheimer's in America

THE SHRIVER REPORT™
on Women and Alzheimer's

A Study by Maria Shriver and
the Alzheimer's Association

Edited by
Karen Skelton, Angela Geiger, Olivia Morgan,
Roberta Hollander and Kathryn Meyer

with
Dale Fetherling and Matt Hickey

Photography by Barbara Kinney

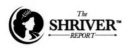

FREE PRESS
New York   London   Toronto   Sydney

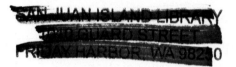
*f*P

Free Press
A Division of Simon & Schuster, Inc.
1230 Avenue of the Americas
New York, NY 10020

First Free Press trade paperback edition April 2011

FREE PRESS and colophon are trademarks of Simon & Schuster, Inc.

For information about special discounts for bulk purchases,
please contact Simon & Schuster Special Sales at 1-866-506-1949
or business@simonandschuster.com

The Simon & Schuster Speakers Bureau can bring authors to your live event.
For more information or to book an event contact the Simon & Schuster Speakers Bureau
at 1-866-248-3049 or visit our website at www.simonspeakers.com.

Manufactured in the United States of America

1 3 5 7 9 10 8 6 4 2

ISBN 978-1-4516-3987-2
ISBN 978-1-4516-2899-9 (ebook)

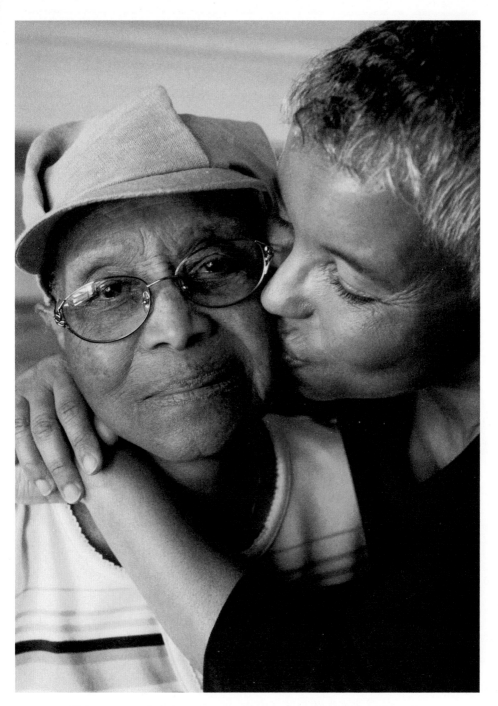

Violette Peters, 53, is the primary caregiver for her mother, Ablyne Winge, 93, who was diagnosed with Alzheimer's disease seven years ago.

Introduction to an Epidemic

By John D. Podesta

O ne look at the numbers on Alzheimer's disease in America shows that the impact on women is both significant and under-examined. Nearly 10 million American women are either suffering from Alzheimer's or caring for someone who is. Family members suffer alongside those afflicted with the disease and often stretch emotional and financial resources to care for their loved ones. In each of these families, it's likely that a woman provides the majority of care. By 2050, the number of women afflicted or caring for someone with Alzheimer's will have more than tripled as the baby boomer generation ages.

That's why *The Shriver Report on Women and Alzheimer's* looks at the epidemic through the eyes of women. The vast majority of caretakers in America are women; often, they bear primary responsibility for raising the next generation as they care for the last. But for the first time in American history, women now also make up half the work force, and two-thirds of all mothers are primary or co-breadwinners in their families. With American women juggling so many responsibilities already, caring for a loved one with Alzheimer's disease can become a Herculean challenge.

This new report builds upon the first, in which Maria Shriver and the Center for American Progress examined the consequences of women comprising half of all U.S. workers. In that groundbreaking study, *The Shriver Report: A Woman's Nation Changes Everything*, we examined this fundamental transformation in the way America works and lives, and how, too often, public policy remains out of step with the needs of modern American families. Above all, *The Shriver Report* detailed the progress women have made in becoming an indispensible and permanent driver of the American economy.

With our partners the Rockefeller Foundation, *Time* magazine, NBC News and others, we ignited an ongoing conversation across the political divide, from the White House and Congress to neighborhoods, conference rooms and kitchen tables across the nation. Following its release, *The Shriver Report* prompted opinion pieces in *The New York Times* and *The Los Angeles Times*, was featured on *NBC Nightly News* and *ABC World News* and generated thousands of news articles, blog posts and online forums. Several universities incorporated *The Shriver Report* as mandatory classroom reading, and people from

140 countries visited our sites to access the report online. And the response we received from men and women leaders in business, government, media, faith communities and, of course, everyday citizens, who recognized the stories in the report in their own lives, was tremendous.

I wrote at the time that "When we look back over the 20th century and try to understand what's happened to workers and their families and the challenges they now face, the movement of women out of the home and into paid employment stands out as a unique and powerful transformation." The truth of this statement will become even more apparent as time passes.

But *The Shriver Report* also underscored the stress, strain and sacrifice American workers endure—and the stark gaps in our societal support structures that, if filled, could help relieve some of these hardships. We wrote about the powerful economic engine women have become in the United States, yet we also pointed out the many obstacles that still keep women from realizing their full potential to contribute to the strength of the American economy.

One finding of the report that resonated in particular was that women's role in the home is as busy as ever. Millions of women play a dual role as both breadwinner and caretaker, putting in 40 or more hours of work outside the home while providing the vast majority of child and family care. Men are increasingly stepping up to the plate, but moms are still juggling the myriad responsibilities of this dual role in a society whose institutions have yet to catch up with modern family life.

And in this second *Shriver Report*, we see that women also provide the bulk of elder care, helping their parents and friends cope with the slow onset of aging and its associated conditions. Some 11.2 million Americans provide billions of hours of unpaid care to people with Alzheimer's or other dementia, and the majority of these caregivers are women. As Maria Shriver so poignantly describes, caring for a parent suffering from Alzheimer's disease—or any of the many illnesses that accelerate and complicate aging—comes at a huge emotional, financial and spiritual toll to oneself and one's family.

As America's 78 million baby boomers enter their 60s, families will confront age-related diseases with increasing frequency. Guided by Maria Shriver's cultural scalpel and relentless intellect, *The Shriver Report on Women and Alzheimer's* will look through the lens of this wasting disease at working women who provide the majority of care to aging friends and family. As we did in our previous study, Maria's new report examines how institutions can keep pace with the realities of the modern family at another transformational moment in American life. And like our first report, this one too will prove to be equally consequential to our understanding of ourselves and our families in this new American era.

John D. Podesta
President and Chief Executive Officer
Center for American Progress

Contents

CONTENTS

Alzheimer's in America

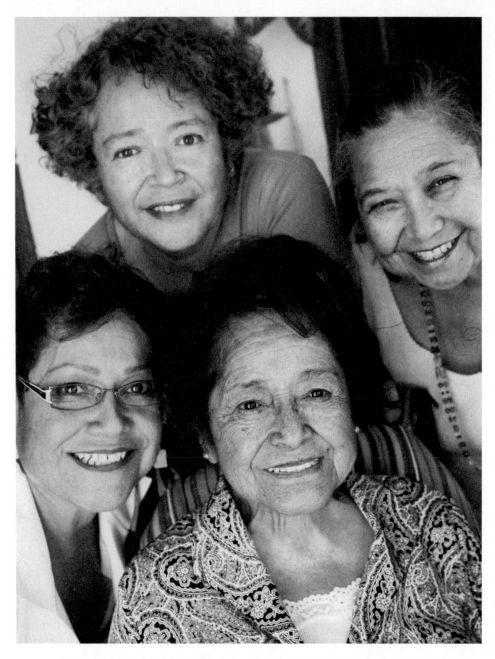

Teresa Rodriguez, top left, Patricia Chavez, top right, and Lisa Parrilla, bottom left, are members of the family care team for their mom, Lupe Rodriguez, 86.

Overview

By Karen Skelton and Angela Timashenka Geiger

*T*he *ShriverReport on Women and Alzheimer's* describes an epidemic of huge proportions for which American women, government, business and families are ill-prepared. Our leaders—and all Americans—need to know the facts.

Most everyone knows *something* about Alzheimer's. Or *knows someone* with the disease. Alzheimer's is quickly taking center stage—hundreds of clinical trials are under way, hundreds of Alzheimer research papers are being published every year, and media coverage occurs almost daily. But what most Americans don't realize—and what this groundbreaking report makes clear—is that women are at the epicenter of Alzheimer's disease.

Never before has a report made such a compelling connection between Alzheimer's disease and women. Sixty-five percent of all those with Alzheimer's are women. Sixty percent of caregivers for persons with Alzheimer's are women. That's 3.3 million American women with Alzheimer's and another 6.7 million women providing care for a friend or loved one. If you consider by mid-century that as many as 8 million women will have Alzheimer's disease, it's clear a huge Alzheimer tsunami is coming at this nation's women. This report is for you.

Why this report?

The Shriver Report on Women and Alzheimer's sounds the alarm for Americans—women, men, government leaders, corporations, nonprofits, churches and the press—to understand that almost a third of Americans have a family member with Alzheimer's and that women are effectively a gender under siege by this disease.

Other reports on Alzheimer's exist. But this one—backed by an extensive, scientific poll, buttressed by in-depth chapters by experts and salted with dozens of poignant, revealing essays and original photography commissioned exclusively for this report—is the first to underscore the impact of the disease on women and how that impact is compounded by the increased risk women have of developing the disease.

What does it show?

The numbers the report reveals are shocking:

- 10 million women either have Alzheimer's or are caring for someone with it.

- Women constitute about two-thirds of those who suffer from Alzheimer's and also about 60 percent of the caregivers for those who have it.

- A third of women caregivers are caring 24/7 for a person with Alzheimer's. Nearly 40 percent say they had no choice in becoming a caregiver.

- The societal impact of Alzheimer's disease—on government, families and business— totals about $300 billion per year.

- Almost two-thirds of all working caregivers report having to go to work late, leave early or take time off to provide care. Yet they get less support for elder care than they do for child care. So it's not surprising that nearly half of all women caregivers report high emotional and physical stress.

Last year, *The Shriver Report: A Woman's Nation Changes Everything* revealed a major tipping point: Working women have emerged as primary breadwinners for millions of households as their presence has grown to comprise fully half of all workers. This new report makes it clear that women are in the midst of an even more far-reaching transfor-mation in which they work, raise kids, care for the elderly, drive consumer decisions and may suffer emotional and physical stress because of it all.

The impact of Alzheimer's is stunning on a broader scale as well. The economic cost, as the report shows, is now about $300 billion a year and could triple in coming decades. As Maria Shriver points out, with 78 million baby boomers now moving into their later years, the cost of Alzheimer's to American society is expected to be $20 trillion between now and 2050. And while annual per-patient costs of Alzheimer's is $56,800, the lion's share of these costs, 60 percent, is borne by families.

Note: With a growing number of people developing Alzheimer's, the number of people impacted and costs related to the disease are constantly changing. For up-to-date Alzheimer's disease statistics visit alz.org.

What needs to be done?

While there's hope and while many researchers are working together feverishly, there's yet no cure or prevention for Alzheimer's. A great deal of fear exists among rank-and-file Americans about developing the disease, and a strong sense pervades the public that not enough scientific progress is being made. Compared to how much progress people believe is being made in combating heart disease, cancer, diabetes and strokes, Americans rank Alzheimer's dead last. So, while there's a lot being done in clinics, research labs and the media to bring Alzheimer's from the shadows to the news, what is not being done is—or should be—making changing the trajectory of Alzheimer's disease a true national priority.

Government, business and citizens themselves must prepare for a future in which Alzheimer's looms larger in American life. Among the key questions that need to be asked and answered:

- How do we get to an appropriate level of public research funding for Alzheimer's, given its high prevalence and cost, both of which are expected to soar?

- Is there a way to reduce the financial impact of the disease on families and society?

- How can we help millions of women caught between the dual demands of work and providing for a friend or relative with Alzheimer's?

- How can average Americans prepare for the very real possibility of Alzheimer's crashing into their lives? Nearly three-quarters (72 percent) say they haven't considered their care options.

- How can government, business, nonprofits and the press effectively call attention to the threat and implement solutions?

In short, as a society we need to do a much better job of keeping pace with the stark realities of Alzheimer's, especially the reality of the besieged American woman who is raising our next generation while caring for our last.

Early-Stage Alzheimer's: "The Fear Is Losing Yourself"

By Mary Ann Becklenberg,
a retired family therapist who lives in Dyer, Indiana

I was diagnosed three years ago at age 62 with early-stage Alzheimer's disease.

I have a master's degree in social work from the University of Chicago, and I worked as a family therapist. The majority of my career was spent in end-stage hospice work, which I dearly loved. I had a lot of responsibilities and always met them and was never overwhelmed by them. All of a sudden—but it wasn't all of a sudden, of course—I began to realize that I wasn't the gal I used to be. It was different inside my head.

It was the very simple things. I would be talking with someone on the telephone, then hang up and ask myself, "Who was that? What did we talk about?" The people in my workplace were saying things like, "See you this afternoon at the meeting at three, Mary Ann." I had no clue that I had missed meetings, and so they began to care for me. My husband says he was shocked and knew something serious was going on when we returned from a vacation together, and I told him, "I really had a great time in California. I'm so sorry you couldn't make it."

It's terribly important to know that you have the disease. If you know, then you don't feel that you're crazy, falling apart, inadequate and terrified. You know that you have a serious disease.

My world as I knew it has irrevocably changed. When I was working, I had introduced a new program to our community called Transitions for individuals who were newly diagnosed with terminal conditions. I helped families meet challenges they had never anticipated. Now I meet challenges myself every day that I had never anticipated. It's not just that I had to leave my beloved work and the self-esteem it provided. I walk with—and work with—the depression and grief experienced by all who share this diagnosis.

More important, my beloved husband, John, has become my caregiver, day in and day out. I'm married to the world's gentlest, most supportive man. We've had the usual ups and downs and challenges that every marriage goes through, but it's no longer a marriage of equals.

It isn't easy being married to me. I'm not always cheerful and dancing around, I can't find things, and I don't remember the sequence. So John picks up the slack. John "co-keeps" my calendar and lovingly anticipates my needs. He is the navigator and coordinator of my day-to-day life. He's rarely short with me, but I'm often short with him—which is not because of him but because of my own frustration with my own self. So one of the challenges is to keep humor in our lives, to laugh about the things you forget. Our three wonderful adult children also provide laughter and love that warm my heart and bring tears to my eyes.

> ❝ My husband says he knew something serious was going on when we returned from a vacation together, and I told him, 'I really had a great time in California. I'm so sorry you couldn't make it.' ❞

The umbrella overarching my new self—my new life—is the Alzheimer's Association. My participation on the Early Stage Advisory Group has been a blessing and a gift. A while ago, they hosted a group of people with Alzheimer's. It was quite an experience because it was actually joyful. It was joyful because you knew that they knew. We didn't have to ask each other how it was that we came to be there. We didn't have to ask, "How's your marriage?" We didn't have to ask, "How is it with your children?"

I cherish the opportunities the Alzheimer's Association gives me to tell my story. I cherish it in my heart, which does not know memory loss. I hope my experience will encourage others to seek early diagnosis when confronted with significant changes in memory that impact daily functioning.

My message to people with Alzheimer's is this: Be gentle with yourself. This disease requires that you lower your expectations of yourself. That's a hard thing for most of us to do. The fear is losing yourself, knowing that you won't bring this self to the end stage of your life. So l look to build my spirit.

When I'm afraid or down or angry or frustrated, I go outside, whatever the weather, and I pray. I believe in a loving God, and I believe in a purpose for life. So I pray a lot. I say, "Come on now, can we move on?" I say to the good Lord, "We've been in this place. Now show me the way and teach me, Lord. Teach me to be gentle with myself."

Working Full-Time, Caregiving Full-Time, Tired Full-Time

By Laura Suihkonen Jones,
a Florida-based training consultant in the aviation software business

*M*y life is a big secret.

I'm a caregiver to my 53-year-old husband, who suffers from Alzheimer's. I'm also a caregiver to my 7-year-old daughter and even occasionally to my 22-year-old son, who is out on his own. I also work full-time.

My secret is how it all affects me. I'm tired, so tired. And I'm terrified. But I fight on because I have no choice.

I do love my job. But working full-time to support my family is hard for me. I just can't make the kind of money my husband did. But how can I increase my earnings when I can't do the job I know I would do if I didn't have Alzheimer's putting roadblocks in my way? I pray I can keep the house, so I don't disrupt my family with the wrenching emotions of moving. People with Alzheimer's don't like to move.

> *66 I'm tired, so tired. And I'm terrified.*
> *But I fight on because I have no choice. 99*

I know I'm very lucky. The nature of my job allows me to deal with family emergencies quietly. I don't want anyone to know I was up all night because my husband was agitated. It's my problem, not theirs. I don't want anyone to know how hard it is for me to show up on time or to know it costs me $16 an hour to have someone watch my family if I have to work late. The emergencies, the fatigue, the stress—it all affects my ability to work. But I don't want to seem like I can't handle it all. Sometimes I let the fear get to me, and then I worry, "If I can't handle it and the job, too, won't I get fired?"

I want my husband back. I need him more than ever now, but he's gone. I can't go to him for advice. I can't go to him for emotional support. He is just like a child. He is egocentric, can't comprehend my feelings, can't remember what I've been doing. In fact, he asks me most mornings what I will do the rest of the day. When I tell him I have to go to work, he is surprised—or sometimes he's angry, because it means I won't be there for him. I want someone to hold me and ease my fears like he used to. Or at least I want him to know that I'm a person like he is. But he doesn't seem to get it anymore.

My body is a wreck. I have gained weight. I have hormonal issues, my blood pressure is up, and I hurt all over. I have asthma and allergies. But my biggest foe is the chronic back pain. I want to have the surgery, but who will watch my family and help me? And where would I get the time? I've already taken double the sick and vacation days I'm allowed for the year.

> **66** *I want my husband back. I need him more than ever now, but he's gone. I can't go to him for advice. I can't go to him for emotional support. He's just like a child.* **99**

Escape is tempting, and I fight the thought every day—escape via food, alcohol and occasionally even the idea of running away, to force someone else to step in. But I won't.

I'm dealing with Alzheimer's disease. There is no hope that it will get better. It will keep getting worse. It will keep getting harder. It will keep costing more money. I will keep doing what I'm doing. And then he will die. I pray that I stay strong so that when he is gone, I don't blame him for my failures or hate myself because I disrespected him in any way.

My husband has Alzheimer's, and I have secrets. Keeping all my secrets requires energy. It's energy I don't have to spare.

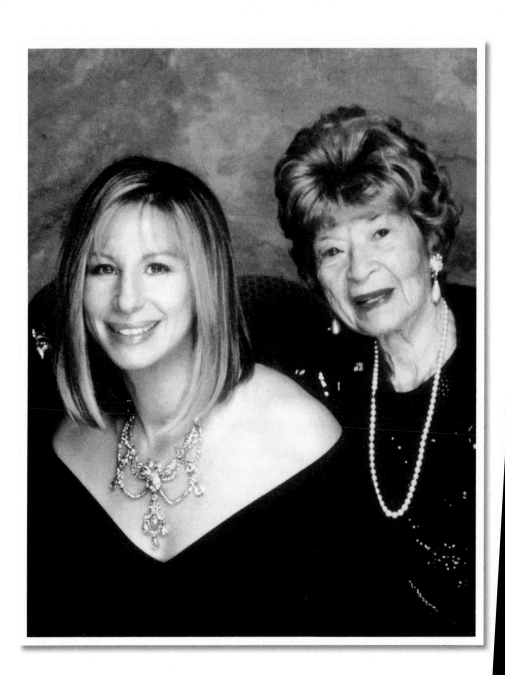

Photo courtesy of Barbra Streisand

Songs She Liked to Sing

*F*or so many years, my mother and I had a difficult relationship. Two strong person-

alities, with plenty of friction between us. But her Alzheimer's erased all that. What's

interesting is that she couldn't remember people or experiences, but she could remember

tunes, songs she liked to sing. My mother had a beautiful voice, and that was probably

the closest we ever were, humming songs together. It's amazing the impact of music on

the brain.

—Barbra Streisand

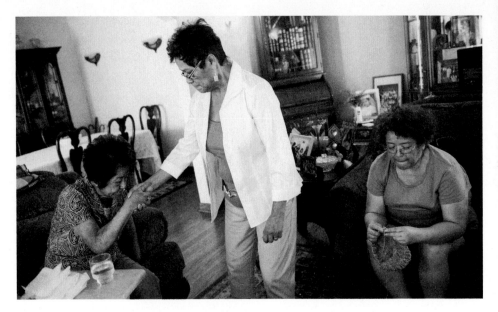

Lisa Parrilla, center, and Teresa Rodriguez, right, are family caregivers for their mother, Lupe Rodriguez, who is living with Alzheimer's disease.

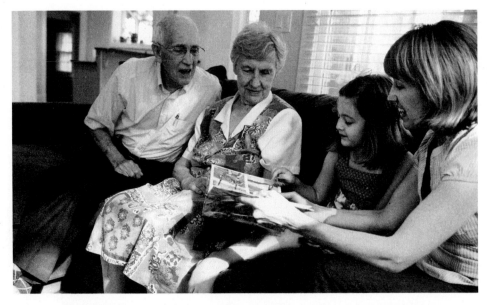

Kaitlin McDowell, 7, shares photos with her grandfather Eugene Kahle, grandmother Kathleen Kahle and mom, Nancy McDowell. Kathleen has been living with Alzheimer's disease for five years.

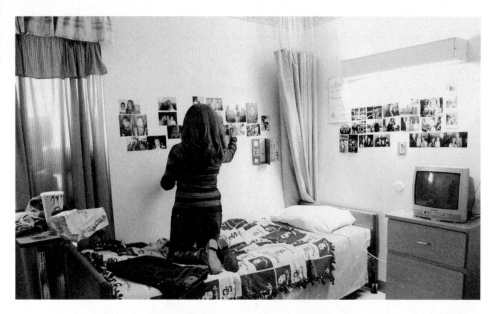

Lindsey Jordan, 16, decorates her father's room at Golden State Care Center in Chatsworth, California. She is one of his primary caregivers.

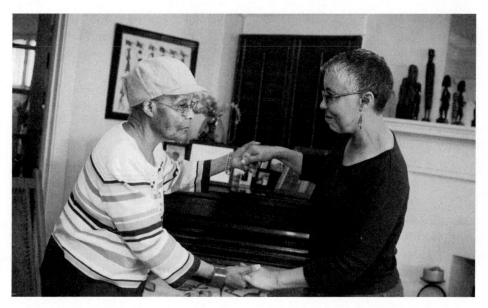

Ablyne Winge goes through her morning routine with her daughter, Violette Peters.

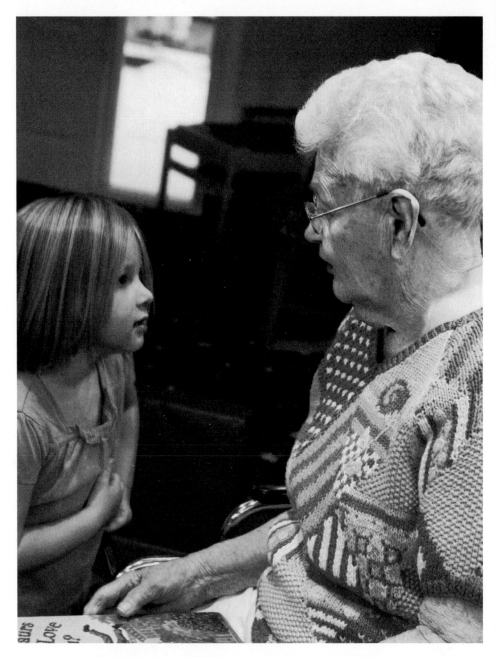

A resident of Lutheran Home in Arlington Heights, Illinois, living with Alzheimer's disease participates in an intergenerational program held at the facility.

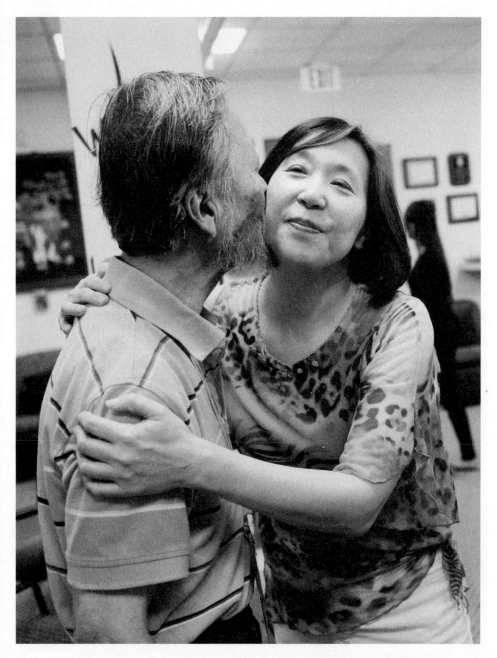

Charles Kao shows his affection for Ruby Ai during adult day care at Catholic Charities Day Break II in Northern California. Charles, who is living with Alzheimer's, was a 2009 Nobel Prize winner in physics.

A Woman's Disease

A Woman's Nation Takes on Alzheimer's

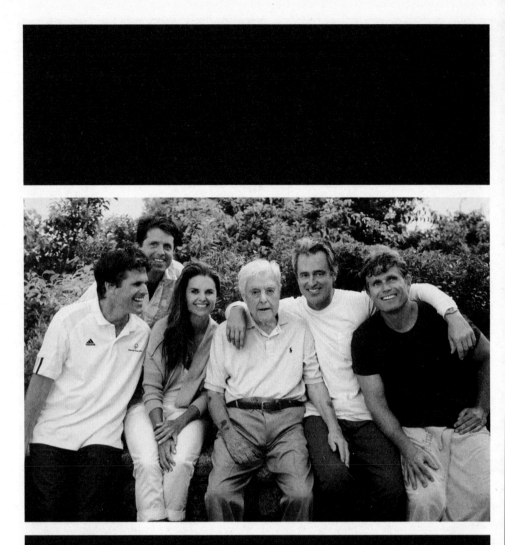

Timothy Shriver, Mark Shriver, Maria Shriver, Sargent Shriver, Bobby Shriver, Anthony Shriver

Photo courtesy of AL Studio, August 2010.

CHAPTER 1

A Woman's Nation Takes on Alzheimer's

By Maria Shriver

I'm Maria Shriver, and I'm a child of Alzheimer's.

That's how I introduced myself last year when I testified before the Senate Special Committee on Aging. I was there to support the Alzheimer's Study Group, a blue-ribbon panel Congress had charged, at the request of the Alzheimer's Association, with designing an action plan to deal with Alzheimer's disease.

Alzheimer's is an epidemic. Every minute or so—in fact, before you get to the end of this page—someone in this country will develop Alzheimer's. Millions of people already have been formally diagnosed. Millions more are undiagnosed—or diagnosed with some form of dementia that could actually be Alzheimer's. And with the 78 million baby boomers now moving into their later years, the cost of Alzheimer's to American society is expected to be $20 trillion between now and the year 2050.[1] That's right—$20 *trillion.*

There's no doubt about it. We are in the midst of a national emergency, and we're woefully unprepared.

So there I was in that packed hearing room, sitting with Alzheimer's Study Group members—former House Speaker Newt Gingrich, former Senator Bob Kerrey, former Supreme Court Justice Sandra Day O'Connor (who had left the High Court to care for her husband with Alzheimer's) and Larry Butcher, chairman of Alzheimer's Community Care in Florida (who would lose his wife months later to younger-onset Alzheimer's). We were all there to ask this powerful congressional committee to listen up, pay attention, increase funding and take on Alzheimer's.

June 12, 2003

Dear Good Friend:

Please forgive this impersonal correspondence, but time is of the essence! After all, I will turn 88 later this year and on June 22nd, I will retire from what has been a full time position for me, -- Chairman of Special Olympics International. Who knows when the next assignment, if any, might be?

Together with Eunice, whose courage and vision started Special Olympics, I have been given over 35 years of unrivalled joy from the athletes, families, volunteers and staff of this remarkable movement.

My extraordinary son, Timothy, has organized and run Special Olympics the past eight years and has brought so much hope, achievement and leadership to our international Special Olympics Program. All of our five children have always worked year in and year out to expand Special Olympics. And they have succeeded!

The joy, the challenge, and the results of Special Olympics are one of the reasons I consider myself to be "the luckiest man on earth." While I will step down from my formal responsibilities, I will never stop doing my part to encourage the world to see the miraculous power of what Eunice has given to all of us. Her creation, "Special Olympics", has given me pleasure and fulfillment beyond description, and I will be grateful for as long as I live.

Nevertheless, it is time to start a new chapter, and at 87, I'm hoping I still have a few chapters left! For all these years, I have done my best to challenge others. Now, I want to challenge myself! I want to keep my ideas fresh so I can actively take part in public debate.

But as we all come to learn sooner or later, desire is only part of the equation. To play a role, one needs not only desire, but skills too; not only a vision, but the ability to put it into action; not only a willingness to work tirelessly, but the friends and allies who together can create the results that make a difference. All of these, I have had, but time has brought unwelcome news too, and for me, it's been tough to accept. Recently, the doctors told me that I have symptoms of the early stages of Alzheimer's Disease! From my point of view, this disease means one thing, and one thing only: my memory is poor. It's a handicap, and it's a challenge. But it does not mean that I am ready to stop challenging myself, or you.

So here's my plan for the coming months: --

First, over recent years, I have begun writing my biography. My last draft was 1,980 typewritten pages, and while I loved every page of it, I realize it needs to be edited! I hope to work on it intensively so that it will be a concise and reliable summary of my life and its lessons. Even if no one else reads it, I'm hoping that Eunice will!

Second, I will work to have my thoughts voiced in journals and magazines of religion and politics. My hope is to contribute from time to time to those magazines and publications which I have read and learned from all of my life. I have no doubt that the world needs to be challenged again—challenged to search for the pathways to peace, challenged to overcome the horrors of poverty and neglect in this country and around the world, challenged to build the international institutions of cooperation that we failed to build in the 20th Century. Hopefully, I can join others in calling on our leaders to do better. I know in my heart that we can.

Third, I hope to devote some significant energy to oral and written remembrances of the personal side of my life: -- of growing up in Westminster and Union Mills, Maryland; of the people and institutions in my home state that helped lay the ground work for my career; of my years in Yale College and Yale Law School, and of the unique and gratifying years as part of some of the great movements of the last half of the 20th Century.

Finally, I hope to have more time to spend with all 15 of my wonderful grandchildren, who are scattered between California, Florida, and Maryland. Eunice, of course, is busier than ever—with political issues, with Special Olympics, with Best Buddies, and with countless campaigns that demand dignity for people with mental retardation. I would gladly scrap any work of my own simply to watch her in action! Age has neither dimmed her anger at injustice nor her humor in overcoming any obstacles the foolhardy throw across her path. What a joy to be part of her whirlwind!

I look forward to being in touch with as many of you as possible. If names are slow to come to me, please forgive me. But if at any moment, I seem content with things as they are, don't leave the room. Remind me of the great times we've had and of the great work waiting to be done. I'm sure I'll be eager to rise to face new challenges, whatever they may be.

All the best,

Sarge

Sargent Shriver

I must admit it was something of a surreal experience for me, because the truth is, for so many years it was my father, Sargent Shriver, who would be sitting in that chair, pleading with senators to listen up, pay attention and increase funding. My dad was the one who would go up to the Hill to testify for his beloved Peace Corps and for all the War On Poverty programs he started and fought for, including Head Start, Vista, Job Corps and Legal Services for the Poor. My father was legendary for the way he worked the Capitol. He knew every senator and congressman by name. He knew their careers, their interests, their politics and their soft spots. He was a brilliant, idealistic and optimistic public servant. My dad was sharp and witty, a walking encyclopedia—his mind a beautifully tuned instrument that left people in awe and inspired.

That was then. Today he doesn't know I'm his daughter, and he doesn't even know my name. To be honest, it's still really difficult to wrap my own mind around that. But so goes the reality and the heartbreak of Alzheimer's. It's a mind-blowing disease—not just for the people who get it, but for everyone around them. That's why I'm so passionate about defeating it.

> *As one of my dad's doctors told me, "Once you've seen one case of Alzheimer's, you've seen...one case of Alzheimer's."*

When my dad was first diagnosed in 2003, my mother, four brothers and I all felt we were entering a world that was confusing, dark and depressing. People just didn't talk about it when Alzheimer's hit their families. They whispered about it, a diagnosis shrouded in shame. There was little information and even less hope.

We struggled to learn about medication and caregiving. We wrestled with handling our father's diminishing independence. How would we explain to him he couldn't drive anymore? How would we tell him he could no longer engage in one of his favorite pastimes, giving rousing speeches about the joys and rewards of public service? When the invitations came in, we'd just send his regrets.

I understand that when people look at Alzheimer families like ours from the outside, they often see dependent parents now cared for by their own offspring, and it seems like the parent-child roles are simply reversed. Not so. The truth is, you hardly feel like you're the parent. You still feel like the helpless child. Even though your father or mother can't work, can't live alone and is as needy as a toddler, you don't feel in control or in charge. No matter who you are, how old you are, what you've accomplished, what your financial situation is—when you're dealing with a parent who has Alzheimer's, you feel powerless. And as the disease unfolds, you feel ever more powerless, because you don't know what to do or what to expect.

As one of my dad's doctors told me, "Once you've seen one case of Alzheimer's, you've seen…one case of Alzheimer's."

In fact, there was so little information back when my Dad was diagnosed that I wrote a book called *What's Happening to Grandpa?* At the time, I said I did it to help my own and other children understand what was going on. In truth, I wrote it to explain Alzheimer's to myself. After it came out, I noticed very few people came up to me to talk about it, because of the stigma still attached to the disease. And when I wanted to put on my broadcast journalist's hat and shine a brighter light on it by turning the book into a TV special, no one was interested. I was told Alzheimer's was a downer and would make for what they called "bad TV." They said Alzheimer's wasn't big enough. It was just "an old person's disease."

Then almost out of nowhere came what I call The Alzheimer's Turning Point. That was March, 21, 2007, when *The New York Times* reported new Alzheimer's Association statistics showing the number of people with Alzheimer's was ballooning—rising by 10 percent in just the previous five years.[2] They reported that fully 13 percent of Americans had Alzheimer's—which meant one in eight people over the age of 65—and unless a cure was found, there would be more than 13 million people with Alzheimer's by 2050, the best guess back then.[3]

That was the wakeup call the baby boomers heard. After all, we were the generation that believed ourselves to be so smart and savvy, that we were very sure our brainspan would match our lifespan. But now, just as the oldest boomers were entering their 60s, these new numbers meant we were at the leading edge of a tsunami—and it was happening not to some nameless old "them" out there. The surge was headed for us, too. And that, I believe, scared a lot of people right out of denial.

It seemed to me that all of a sudden, Alzheimer's became front-page news and people really started paying attention. That's when HBO came to me and said, "We want to take an in-depth look into Alzheimer's disease, and we want you to be involved."

So, starting on Mother's Day last year, HBO aired the most comprehensive television event about the disease ever, *The Alzheimer's Project.* There were four broadcasts and a companion book covering in great depth the cutting-edge science, the issue of caregiving, what it's like to have the disease and the impact on the children and grandchildren of Alzheimer's. Along with HBO's legendary Sheila Nevins, I co-executive produced this massive project. All of a sudden, everywhere I went people approached me to voice their fears, share their experience and ask for advice. "The Alzheimer's Project" won several Emmys. It attracted 11 million viewers when it aired, and people are still watching all four parts of it at www.hbo.com/alzheimers/the-films.html.

About the same time last year, I was working on the very first *The Shriver Report: A Woman's Nation Changes Everything.* It was a landmark study—published in collaboration with the Center for American Progress—exploring a transformational moment in the United States. It arose from my work as First Lady of California, where I've helmed The Women's Conference, the biggest forum for women in the nation.

The transformational moment was this: For the first time in our nation's history, women were becoming the majority of the workforce—and also primary or co-breadwinners in almost two-thirds of American families.[4] We were now what I called A Woman's Nation. I knew this shift would impact every institution in our country: the family, the workplace, the healthcare system, government services, even the relationship between men and women themselves.

More than 40 percent of women said that they were the main caregivers for elderly parents.

What came out of that report—its studies, analyses, essays by cultural leaders and a huge, groundbreaking nationwide opinion survey—was the first comprehensive and accurate portrait of The Way Things Are Now in the American home and workplace. It was also the first accounting of exactly how out of step our institutions are with the needs of women today.

We learned that women aren't just primary breadwinners. They're still the primary caregivers in their families as well. Almost 70 percent of the women we surveyed for the first *Shriver Report* told us that despite working full-time, they're still the ones most responsible for taking care of the children.[5] More than 40 percent of them said that they were the main caregivers for elderly parents.[6] And almost a third of them said they were primary caregivers of both their kids and their parents.[7]

We wondered whether their employers were adjusting, offering help like child care and flexible hours. You'd think so, because studies show that when "employees have greater access to flexible work arrangements, they are more committed and loyal to their employers and are willing to work harder than required to help their employers be successful."[8] Yet we found that so many companies and institutions were simply out of touch with workers' needs today.

We held roundtables around the country, where women who knew I was dealing with four kids, my own sick mother and a father with Alzheimer's would come up to me and say, "Me, too! I'm in the same boat, and I need help!"

Bingo! That's when I realized that Alzheimer's was emerging as another huge transformational force exerting a powerful pressure on women, families and our institutions. Alzheimer's was in the process of changing A Woman's Nation forever.

- Today, women are not only a dominant economic force in this country. They also make up 65 percent of the people with Alzheimer's—and up to three-fifths of all Alzheimer caregivers are women as well.[9]

This perfect storm made me realize it was time for another *Shriver Report*, this time in partnership with the Alzheimer's Association.

In addition to an in-depth examination of the issues and trends by experts—and searingly honest personal essays by people from every walk of life affected by Alzheimer's, including several women who have the disease—we have conducted an enormous nationwide survey of 3,118 adults, including more than 500 Alzheimer caregivers. Our findings show the huge impact of Alzheimer's behind closed doors in this country:

- Almost 90 percent of Americans who know someone with the disease are concerned that they or someone close to them will get Alzheimer's.

- Half of women caring for someone with Alzheimer's are providing more than 40 hours a week of care. A third of women caregivers care for their loved one 24/7.

- Nearly 41 percent of the women caregivers said they had no choice in taking care of their loved one with Alzheimer's.

- More than half of the family caregivers of people with Alzheimer's we surveyed said it's straining their family finances.

- Nearly 65 percent of working caregivers of people with Alzheimer's told us they need to come to work late, leave early or take time off from their jobs as a result of their caregiving responsibilities.

- Nearly a third of women caregivers rate the physical stress level of caregiving a 5 out of 5.

- The greatest fears women voice about getting Alzheimer's is that they will forget their loved ones, become a burden to their families and not be able to care for themselves.

My hope is that this *Shriver Report* triggers another Alzheimer's Turning Point and gets the national conversation focused on this disease and its ramifications. It's time. We must face up to some big questions: With Americans living longer and with the incidence of Alzheimer's growing, what's going to happen to our women, our families, our workplaces, our attitudes, our society, as the Alzheimer wave hits over the next few decades? We're talking crisis.

Doctors and researchers at the National Institute on Aging and the Alzheimer's Association are now looking into the possibility of revising how and when they diagnose Alzheimer's. They've begun the long process of reviewing what they call "the diagnostic criteria" for the disease.[10]

Why the review? Well, until now, Alzheimer's has been diagnosed only when clinical symptoms are apparent. This means significant damage is already done in the brain, such as the telltale plaques and tangles so long considered the definitive sign of Alzheimer's. But now, better diagnostic tools like MRIs and brain scans and spinal taps looking for specific biomarkers could mean that doctors might one day be able to detect changes in the living brain much earlier—years before there are even any signs of dementia.

But any possible revision of the way Alzheimer's is diagnosed is still a long way off. And until then, some researchers are warning about using these very expensive high-tech tests for screening the general population, for two reasons. One, the tests sometimes find plaques in the brains of people who never even develop Alzheimer's. And two, there's no effective treatment or cure for Alzheimer's anyway.[11]

So how many people do we think actually have or will get Alzheimer's disease? Well, until there are new standards for diagnosis, it's unclear. The estimates are all over the map. The actual number of Americans with Alzheimer's disease today may be far more than the official 5.3 million number we all use.[12] And what about the projection that by 2050, there'll be up to 16 million people with Alzheimer's disease in this country?[13] I bet it could turn out to be a bigger number than that.

But whatever the number of cases is, this much we know for sure: Most of them are expected to be women. And most of the people who will end up taking care of them will be women, too.

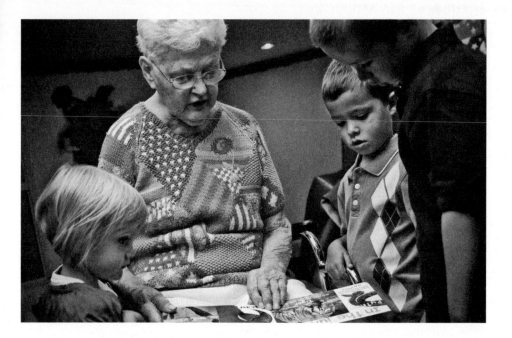

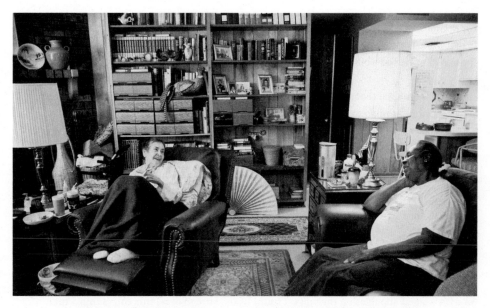

Shirley Carreras of New Orleans chats with one of her caregivers, Gloria Wright. Gloria comes in four partial days a week to provide respite for Shirley's family.

- The President's Council of Economic Advisors reported this year that 43.5 million Americans—most of them women—are providing unpaid caregiving to relatives and friends over the age of 50.[14]

- More specifically, our poll showed that today, the average unpaid Alzheimer caregivers are working women over the age of 50 providing care most commonly to their mothers (31 percent) and spouses (15 percent).

And that unpaid caregiving—which so often comes on top of a paying job and childrearing—is tough physical and emotional work.

- The truth is it's women who are the ones who generally do the hands-on grunt work of caregiving[15]—cleaning their parents or spouses and changing their diapers, feeding them, babysitting them, dispensing medication to them. While men do represent about a third of family caregivers,[16] they tend to arrange or supervise outside services.[17]

For decades, women have fought for respect for mothers and recognition that mothering is real work. Now we have to fight for respect for caregivers and recognition that caregiving is real work, too—billions of dollars worth of work.

- AARP estimated that 34 million caregivers over the age of 18 in the United States provided $375 billion worth of unpaid services a year—more than the yearly state plus federal Medicaid spending—and that was three years ago![18] By the way, add this to the mix: Nearly 1.4 million kids aged 8 to 18 are helping take care of an adult relative[19]—250,000 of them caring for loved ones with Alzheimer's or other dementias.[20]

This Woman's Nation has truly become a Caregiver Nation as well, and Alzheimer's is putting the pedal to the metal. To be specific:

- This year it's estimated there are 11.2 million Alzheimer and other dementia caregivers, and 6.7 million of them are—you guessed it—women.[21]

So with women shouldering the biggest brunt of the burden of all this caregiving, I find it ironic that we're still seeing articles like "Why Aren't Women Happy?" They wonder why women aren't satisfied with their advanced degrees and new corner offices. They ask, "What's Happened to Her Sex Drive?" and "What's Wrong with American Women?" Excuse me?

What's right with American women is that they're rearing and providing for the next generation of Americans, while at the same time caring and providing for the previous generation of Americans. What's right with American women is that they're doing it even though studies show that caregivers pay a steep price in terms of their own health—increased stress, depression, lost sleep, chronic anxiety, immune-system deficiency.[22] They're paying a financial price as well, because full-time workers who are also caregiving at home have lower earning power.[23]

American women are stressed-out and maxed-out. There's nothing wrong with them! They just need support. What has to get right is our institutions. They need to respond to the changing dynamic in the American home. People with Alzheimer's cannot live alone, and the family members who live with them and take care of them need help.

Health and Human Services Secretary Kathleen Sebelius lays out for us in this report many provisions in the 2010 healthcare reform legislation, The Affordable Care Act, that provide relief for Alzheimer's caregivers.

It's a start. But we also need to have a national conversation about what else the growing millions of Alzheimer families need:

- We have a Dependent Care Tax Credit for employment-related child care expenses. But what about a meaningful Elder Care Tax Credit?

- How about incentivizing flextime programs, so employers are really encouraged to offer flexible work hours to their caregiving employees?

- The federal government and some states provide for Maternity Leave and Family Leave. How about Elder Care Leave, including coverage for emergencies at home? Maybe more men would step up and help out at home if they knew taking time off was OK with their employers.

- How about more access to high-quality Alzheimer training for both family members and paid home healthcare aides? How about actually teaching family members how to really stay on top of all the medications they have to dispense?

- How about more elder daycare programs staffed with people actually accredited for Alzheimer care? Believe it or not, less than 1 percent of practicing nurses nationwide are credentialed in gerontology.[24]

- And what about more government quality control of seniors' programs, nursing homes and end-of-life facilities, before we have an epidemic of elder abuse accompanying the rise in Alzheimer's?

- How about more intergenerational daycare centers, like the one I visited in San Diego, where toddlers and people with Alzheimer's spend the day together? They eat together, they dance together, go to storytime together. It's quite moving to behold. And what about more intergenerational playgrounds? We built the first one in California, so Sandwich Generation people like me—taking care of both kids and parents—can go to one place with all of them.

- And how about more governmental support for adult daycare and respite care programs in general, so we can give family caregivers a break now and then?

I know, I know. Let me say it before you do: "Who's gonna pay for all these programs? We're in a recession!" Many states, including my own, are struggling with staggering budget deficits. And many political leaders, including my own husband, are wrestling with cutting many of the same types of programs I'm advocating.

But that's exactly why we need a new kind of national conversation about Alzheimer's and growing old in America—just like the conversations heard around kitchen tables all over the country. Families are sitting down to figure out how to pay for their portion of the billions of dollars of unpaid care elders are receiving at home. American families are asking and answering the same questions we need to ask and answer on a state and national level:

- "How can we afford this care? How can we pay for it?"
- "Whose job is it—whose turn is it—to do the caregiving?"

We need more of us at that kitchen table. Not just the Alzheimer's Association fighting the disease and providing support, but a partnership of families, businesses, faith-based institutions, unions, government leaders, insurance companies, healthcare institutions—everybody on the front lines, all of us accountable. And since personal and family responsibility will always be a huge piece of the Alzheimer's care picture:

- How about Elder Care Savings Plans like the 401K retirement savings plans and 529 college savings plans? Since our parents are living longer, many families could start socking away at least some money now.

If we wait until the crest of the Age Wave hits—and it's coming—it will be too late. It's just like Katrina. If the levees were built strong enough the first time, they would have held.

Of course, our biggest hope for Alzheimer's lies in medical research. As you'll read in this report, we're getting closer, but our scientists are still chipping away at critical questions like these:

- What causes Alzheimer's? Is it inherited? What causes younger-onset Alzheimer's? Is there any treatment that can delay the onset or slow down the course of the disease?

- What about new tests that may be able to tell you if you're going to get Alzheimer's? Are the tests ready for use? Are they accurate? Who would be a candidate to take them? If there are no foolproof treatments yet, what's the good of knowing?

- What can we do to prevent Alzheimer's? Do lifestyle changes really help? Should we all be hitting the treadmill, drinking tea, doing crossword puzzles, taking Omega-3 and Vitamin D?

- Why do more women get Alzheimer's than men? Is it just because women live longer? Does estrogen play a part in prevention? If so, how much and when?

- What exactly is the natural course of the disease? Why does it play out in a few years for some patients, in a decade or more for others? Why do different people have different symptoms: some explosively angry, others hypersexual, still others mumbling or even silent? In other words, why is it that "once you've seen one case of Alzheimer's, you've seen...one case of Alzheimer's"?

- And for God's sake, when will there be a cure?

For HBO's *The Alzheimer's Project,* I visited labs where our brilliant scientists work around the clock, deeply immersed in research they hope will lead to a cure. But while the federal government will spend about $6 billion on cancer research and about $4 billion for research on cardiovascular diseases this coming year, we're investing a fraction of that, less than $500 million a year, on Alzheimer research.[25] The 2010 healthcare reform act could boost that effort some, but it won't be enough.

I've come to believe that brain research is one of the most important investments our country can make, period. I believe the brain is for America today what the moon was for America in the 1960s: The Next Frontier. I'm convinced if we make a national commitment and launch more of our best doctors and scientists at the brain, they'll one day produce treatments and prevention strategies and even cures—not just for Alzheimer's but for a whole host of brain diseases, like Parkinson's disease, Huntington's disease, stroke, dementia, mental illness, Down syndrome, autism, addiction, depression. Unlocking the secrets of the brain will teach us more about who we are, how we work, how we learn, what makes us tick and what makes us sick and how to fix it—so that fewer families will have to go through what my family has gone through because of a devastating brain disease.

Which brings me back to my father.

Several months after my mother's death last year, my four brothers and I wondered what to do with our dad. The house my parents had shared was way too big for him: too lonely, too isolated, too much. We wondered if we should we leave him in Washington or move him to Florida or California to live with one or another of his children.

We need a new kind of national conversation about Alzheimer's and growing old in America.

After much discussion and debate and advice from doctors, we concluded that the best thing for our dad would be to keep him in his neighborhood, down the street from two of my brothers, in a facility with lots of people and activities and full-time medical care. It was an excruciatingly painful decision, as it is for any Alzheimer family who makes it. We called it a "temporary decision," and we'd see how it went.

We sold my parents' home, packed everything up, moved it all out and put my dad into a beautiful assisted living home right down the street. When I went to check it out for the first time, I sat on the floor and burst into tears, unsure whether we were making the right decision. We made his room look exactly like his room at home. I don't think he noticed, but it made us feel better.

I remember the first time I went there to visit him. It was seven years after his diagnosis, mind you, but it felt like I was dealing with his disease head-on for the first time. Why? I realize now that while my mother was alive, I was more focused on her—talking to her every day, dealing her declining health, her strokes, her many emergency hospitalizations. Focusing on her distracted me from really feeling the impact of my dad's disease. Call it what it was: denial. But since she's gone, my dad's Alzheimer's has hit me in the face, and it's cracked my denial wide open.

When I went to visit my father recently in Washington, I took him outside. There we were, three people sitting quietly on a park bench—his caregiver and me, with my dad in the middle. After a while, my father put his head down on the caregiver's shoulder and nuzzled him, just like a little kid. It was a sweet moment, looking as he did like a child seeking and getting comfort. But not from me. It was as if I, his only daughter, weren't there at all. I could have been a bystander. Actually, I was a bystander. That blew my mind and broke my heart.

Today, I visit him and call him, because I know I should. It's the right thing to do. It's the respectful thing to do. It's what a good daughter does. I would want it done for me. But I still struggle. I struggle to find my place in his life and his care, and I struggle for a connection. I say, "Hello, Daddy." He says, "God bless you!" I say, "How are you, Daddy?" He says, "You're fantastic!" Sometimes he just mumbles. Sometimes I don't get even that.

I watch my dad in the facility's day room, playing with the same puzzles and alphabet blocks my kids had when they were 5 years old. Doing the same things we used to do in Mommy 'n' Me classes. I can't even describe what I feel when I see that.

If I want to remember Sargent Shriver, the smartest person I ever knew, the World War II naval hero, the editor of the Yale newspaper, the devoted husband and father, the brilliant and successful public servant with the dazzling intellect—that Sargent Shriver, my dad, is in the pictures on the wall in his room.

I'm so grateful to my brothers and their wives who have homes in Washington down the street from the facility, who step up in such a substantial way to take care of our dad. They have him over for dinner every night and take him to their kids' basketball games and recitals and to church. They are fully present with him. They know how to deal with him and talk to him. When he refuses to get out of the car, my brothers say, "Fine!" When he growls at them, they growl back. When he mumbles, they mumble.

We talk about how women are doing the lion's share of Alzheimer caregiving in this country. But all four of my brothers and men whose stories you'll read in this report show us that men have been stepping up to the plate to care for ailing parents as well. And more men will have to, as more and more women, including their own wives, get the disease. As we investigate in this report, men are having to change their attitudes about what helping out at home means, about asking for flexible work schedules, about how to run their own businesses, how to juggle doctors' appointments, how to manage medications, how to take care of their aging in-laws when their wives can't—how to sit and look into the face of a spouse or parent who doesn't know who on earth they are and deal with it.

It's a tough change for so many of them. We women inhabit caretaking roles easily, and men have said for so long, "I just don't know how to do what you do, and I'm just not as good at it as you are." Now women are asking the men in our lives to help us—and they are.

I watch my four brothers give their kids a new kind of role model to emulate: the strong, nurturing man. My brothers treat my father with such love—fixing his jacket, smoothing his hair, telling him, "Lookin' sharp, Daddy!" One more time, he says, "That's fantastic!" They take him to Orioles and Red Sox games and to Special Olympics and Best Buddies events, where former Peace Corps volunteers come up to see him. They know he has Alzheimer's, but still they take his hand and tell him stories from the old days. It doesn't matter that he doesn't know who they are or that he doesn't even remember the Peace Corps. What matters is that he's comforted by the warmth of the human connection. These are the gifts my brothers bring to him.

And I've learned from my own children and my nieces and nephews. I watch how they talk and laugh with their grandpa, funny and free and easy. They love him, they laugh with him, they play with him, they're fascinated by him. They don't get bogged down in the sadness. My kids and my nieces and nephews all accept my father for who he is today—and that's been a lesson in acceptance for me.

For the summer, we moved our dad out of the facility in Washington to our family home in Hyannis Port. We all took turns living there with him. It felt good and right to be in the same house with him, being next to him at dinner, playing ball with him or just sitting in silence with him, staring out at the sea. I talked to him about my mother, and we looked at old pictures together. When I had to leave to go home to California, I felt guilty and conflicted.

I know that all in all, my family is so lucky. We're truly blessed we have been able to keep our father at home for a long time. We are blessed to have the choices we have today. We're especially blessed to have the resources to pay patient and loving caregivers who help us take care of our dad and make him feel loved.

But I know millions of others aren't as lucky. Many are forced to quit jobs to stay home— or go through the wrenching process of sending a parent away to a facility, feeling judged and mortified and ashamed that they can't care for their loved one themselves. That's the double stigma of Alzheimer's—ashamed that you have it in your family, ashamed that you can't cope. For so many, the financial, emotional and spiritual costs are just way too much to bear.

My hope is that as the veil is lifted, as information and funds and support programs are made available, families will see that they're not alone. As more people, like the ones you'll meet in *The Shriver Report*, step out and speak out, sharing their personal journeys with Alzheimer's, more families will see that there's nothing to be ashamed of—that there's hope out there because, together, we are finally making Alzheimer's a national issue.

The truth is that we simply must put Alzheimer's on the front burner because if we don't, Alzheimer's will not just devour our memories. It will also break our women, cripple our families, devastate our healthcare system and decimate the legacy of our generation.

But if we do, I'm convinced that this Woman's Nation will be able to say that, believe it or not, there once was a time when there was no cure for Alzheimer's.

ENDNOTES

1   *Changing the Trajectory of Alzheimer's Disease: A National Imperative,* Alzheimer's Association 2010.

2   "Prevalence of Alzheimer's Rises 10% in 5 Years", Jane Gross, *New York Times,* March 21, 2007, quoting data from 2007 *Alzheimer's Disease Facts and Figures,* Alzheimer's Association, p. 6.

3   Ibid.

4   *The Shriver Report: A Woman's Nation Changes Everything*: A Study by Maria Shriver and the Center for American Progress, p. 17.

5   Ibid.

6   Ibid.

7   Ruy Teixeira, Center for American Progress, analysis of data from *The Shriver Report: A Woman's Nation Changes Everything,* personal communication.

8   Ibid, p. 219.

9   The 3.3 million figure was provided to the Alzheimer's Association by Denis Evans, M.D., on July 21, 2010. The figure is derived from data published in Hebert LE, et al., "Alzheimer's disease in the U.S. population: Prevalence estimates using the 2000 census," *Archives of Neurology* 2003, 60 : pp.1119–1122. Based on the data, Dr. Evans' research team calculated the number of women age 65 and older with Alzheimer's disease in 2010.

10   Proposed Revisions to Diagnostic Criteria for Alzheimer's Disease, National Institute on Aging and the Alzheimer's Association, July 2010.

11   "Alzheimer's Isn't Up to the Tests," Dr. Sanjay W. Pimplikar, *New York Times* Op-Ed, July 19, 2010.

12   *2010 Alzheimer's Disease Facts and Figures,* Alzheimer's Association, p. 10.

13   Ibid, p. 14.

14   President's Council of Economic Advisers, "Work-life Balance and the Economics of Workplace Flexibility," March 2010, p. 2, quoting National Alliance for Caregiving, *Caregiving in the U.S. : A Focused Look At Those Caring for Someone Age 50 or Older,* November 2009.

15   "Caregiving in the U.S. 2009," op cit, p. 6.

16   Ibid, p. 14.

17   Ibid p. 25.

18   *Valuing the Invaluable: The Economic Caregiving,* 2008 Update, AARP Public Policy Institute, p. 1.

19   Young Caregivers in the U.S., National Alliance for Caregiving and the United Hospital Fund, 2005.

20   *2010 Alzheimer's Disease Facts and Figures 2010,* Alzheimer's Association. p. 26.

21   The 11.2 million figure is based on the estimated number of unpaid caregivers of people with Alzheimer's disease and other dementias in 2009, as shown in *2010 Alzheimer's Disease Facts and Figures* (10.9 million), updated to 2010 by multiplying the 10.9 million figure by the percent increase in the U.S. population age 18 and older from July 2009 to June 2010 (the latest available figure from the U.S. Census), 2.8 percent, and adding that total, 300,000, to 10.9 million.

22   R. Schulz, L.M. Martire, "Family caregiving of persons with dementia: Prevalence, health effects, and support strategies," *American Journal of Geriatric Psychiatry,* 2004, pp. 240–249.

23   The MetLife Juggling Act Study: Balancing Caregiving with Work and the Costs Involved—Findings from a National Study by the National Alliance for Caregiving and the National Center on Women and Aging at Brandeis University, November 1999, p. 5.

24 Claudia Beverly, PhD, RN, "Aging Issues: Nursing Imperatives for Healthcare Reform," *Nursing Administration Quarterly,* April/June 2010, p. 99.

25 National Institutes of Health, *Estimates of Funding for Various Research, Condition, and Disease Categories,* Feb. 1, 2010, http://report.nih.gov/rcdc/categories/PFSummaryTable.aspx.

Lisa Carbo, 56, cares for her mom, Shirley Carreras, 79. Both women are living with Alzheimer's disease.

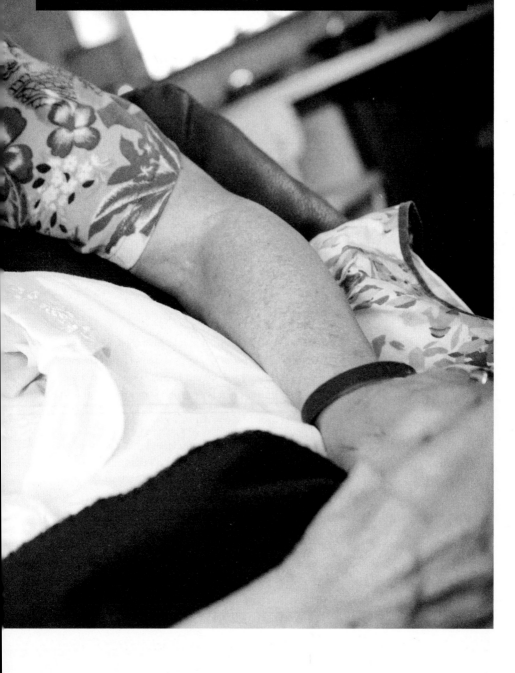

Essays: Daughters Reflect

"We Didn't Know Then What We Know Now"

By Princess Yasmin Aga Khan, president of Alzheimer's Disease International, honorary vice chairman of the national board of the Alzheimer's Association and general chair of the Alzheimer's Association Rita Hayworth Galas

My mother, Rita Hayworth, was the most beautiful and glamorous movie star of the 1940s and 1950s. She spent much of her life memorizing complicated dance routines and movie scripts. How ironic that she would later be diagnosed with Alzheimer's disease.

As a young girl on visits home from boarding school, I would notice her odd behavior. She would move her personal items from her bedroom to other closets around the house, including mine. She would throw all the food out of the cupboards. She would imagine voices outside and think someone was trying to break into her home. The police would have to come and tell her no one was there. I remember the many times she would call me at college and ask me the same questions over and over again.

As the disease progressed, her confusion, disorientation and fear worsened. She was unable to remember what day it was or even the name of our president. Her panic increased, and my own fear and sense of helplessness and guilt became overwhelming. It was a terrible day when we stood together in front of a mirror, and she turned to me and asked, "Who are you?"

It wasn't until she had a complete breakdown that I could step in and take charge of my dear mother's life. I became her caregiver, and I worried about her all the time.

My thought back then was, "What on earth is going on? What's happening to her?" Today, she would be diagnosed with younger-onset Alzheimer's disease, since she was only in her 50s. But this was the 1970s. We didn't know then what we know now. Very few people had heard of Alzheimer's disease, and it was often misdiagnosed. Patients would be over-medicated and some even sent to mental institutions.

The best anyone could come up with was that she was suffering from alcoholic dementia. She did like to drink, but it wasn't that much, and I now believe that alcohol helped her cope with the knowledge that she was losing her memory and, ultimately, her career as well.

At last, in 1981, thanks to Dr. Ronald Fieve—with the help of a CAT scan and memory test—we got the right diagnosis. I felt such a great sense of relief knowing exactly what was wrong. Alzheimer's can be an embarrassing and humiliating disease not just to people who have it but to friends and family as well, and early diagnosis by a neurologist is key to coping.

With the word of my mother's illness getting out, I was approached by the Alzheimer's Association, which had recently been started by Chicago businessman Jerome Stone, whose wife had the disease. This organization was my savior. At that time, the Alzheimer's Association was a small mom-and-pop group made up of husbands, wives, sons and daughters who had family members with the disease. All these wonderful people were my support group. We were there for each other. We shared our daily knowledge and experience of how to best care for our loved ones.

We sprang into action. We went to Washington to push for federal funding for Alzheimer research, because there was very little money spent on the disease at the time. We raised dollars to award to young researchers doing work in the field. We developed Alzheimer's Association chapters around the country to support caregivers and make sure they knew that they were not alone. We participated in the development of Alzheimer's Disease International (ADI), of which there are presently 72 member countries.

We continue our efforts today, pressing for heightened public awareness, increased government engagement, more research dollars, programs providing respite for caregivers and financial relief for those who cannot afford home care attendants and costly nursing homes.

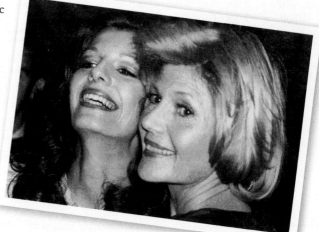

My mother passed away in 1987. We have come a very long way since then. But there is so much more work still to be done.

Photo courtesy of Princess Yasmin Aga Khan

"You Are My Sunshine"

By Kathy Mattea,
Grammy Award–winning country music star

*I*n December 1999, I took my mother, Ruth, to the Mayo Clinic. The doctors there diagnosed her with Alzheimer's disease. They said the average life expectancy after an Alzheimer diagnosis was five years. She died in August 2005, five-and-a-half years later.

We had watched her next-oldest sister go through the process of Alzheimer's. It was excruciating. My mother, who had always been the rock of the family, could hardly stand to go visit. She had too much grief to be able to bear the truth of what was happening to her sister.

The next five years were a roller coaster ride for all of us, with many blessings and many hard days. She went through the various stages—from denial to anger to "You're having an affair!"

There were periods of time where each one of us—each family member and sometimes the caregivers—was "in the dog house." Each would become my mom's scapegoat for her anger when she couldn't express her fear and dread. I believe it was easier for her to feel angry with one of us when she got overwhelmed. I imagine that made her feel like she had some kind of power.

As she moved through the various stages, though, she became softer and softer. The anger began to subside, and we realized we had open access to her sweet, innocent heart. This was the time that we relished most. I remember and cherish many of these small moments, carrying them like beads on a string as my comfort on the days when I miss her beyond words.

I would go home to visit and just sit with her on the couch with her feet in my lap. We'd hold hands, we'd visit, we'd be silly, we'd watch TV. She loved *Law and Order*, her favorite show. And I began to notice that when the commercials came on, she would tap my hand along with the music, something she'd never done before. I loved feeling her connecting to this background music I had long overlooked, and her primal response to it. It gave me a small, sweet surge of joy.

Some time later I went home to visit on my way through to a college reunion. I had ordered a guitar for a friend's son who was getting into playing, and it was delivered to my mom's house. I took it out, tuned it up and hit a chord. And right there on the patio, my mother burst into song.

I was astonished.

You see, my mother was tone deaf. She never sang. She was too shy, too embarrassed. But when she got Alzheimer's, she forgot that she "couldn't" sing, and so she sang all the time.

That day, for the first time in my life, I sang with my mother. I played guitar and we sang all afternoon, and she had such openness and joy. I was comforted by this unexpected connection, especially since any conventional conversation had become impossible by then.

A year later, when she finally didn't know me anymore, she could still sing all the verses to "You Are My Sunshine" with me. It was our last connection—and the memory I hold most dear.

One Woman's Travels
with Alzheimer's

By Patti Davis, who has written eight books, including The Long Goodbye, *dealing with the Alzheimer's disease of her father, former president Ronald Reagan. Her most recent is* The Lives Our Mothers Leave Us.

*T*here is an underlying truth to losing a loved one: Everyone loses that person in their own way. Gender, history, the designs and intricacies of one's emotions—as unique in individuals as the patterns of snowflakes—all play a part. It's particularly true in families. You may be gathered around the same bedside, but at the core of everyone's soul, the experience is solitary and personal.

I can't tell you how my brothers or my mother or my sister Maureen (who died before our father) experienced his slow and inexorable slide into Alzheimer's—a death before death. The disease is a vanishing into the valley of the shadow, and no one else can follow. I can only tell you what it was like for me.

> **66** *Maybe women are a little more willing to live alongside death and dying because, on a cellular level, we understand birth.* **99**

I lost my father as a daughter, with all that that implies. I lost him as a small girl who once gazed up at him and believed he could do anything. I lost him as a teenager who craved more of his attention and came up empty most of the time, who eventually figured out that if she roiled the waters, unleashed enough battle cries, he would have to notice her. Ultimately, I lost him in the softer territory of a woman who had asked his forgiveness but still couldn't quite forgive herself for the wounds she'd inflicted.

I've noticed that women metabolize the reality of death and dying differently from men. Particularly with a disease like Alzheimer's, where parts of a person die off gradually, it's been my observation that men tend to back away in discomfort. During the last years of

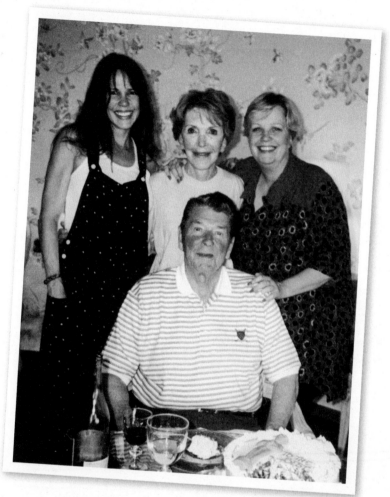

Father's Day 1995

my father's life, I would occasionally run into a high-powered CEO whose mother also had Alzheimer's. He told me he visited her, but not that often or for that long because, in his words, "She doesn't know who I am. She sometimes doesn't even know I'm there. So, there's no point." He was visibly uncomfortable, fidgety even. This was a man who could rule a conference room and make decisions worth millions of dollars. He was known as

RONALD REAGAN

Nov. 5, 1994

My Fellow Americans,

I have recently been told that I am one of the millions of Americans who will be afflicted with Alzheimer's Disease.

Upon learning this news, Nancy & I had to decide whether as private citizens we would keep this a private matter or whether we would make this news known in a public way.

In the past Nancy suffered from breast cancer and I had my cancer surgeries. We found through our open disclosures we were able to raise public awareness. We were happy that as a result many more people underwent testing. They were treated in early stages and able to return to normal, healthy lives.

So now, we feel it is important to share it with you. In opening our hearts, we hope this might promote greater awareness of this condition. Perhaps it will encourage a clearer understanding of the individuals and families who are affected by it.

At the moment I feel just fine. I intend to live the remainder of the years God gives me on this earth doing the things I have always done. I will continue to share life's journey with my beloved Nancy and my family. I plan to enjoy the great outdoors and stay in touch with my friends and supporters.

Unfortunately, as Alzheimer's Disease progresses, the family often bears a heavy burden. I only wish there was some way I could spare Nancy from this painful experience. When the time comes I am confident that with your help she will face it with faith and courage.

In closing let me thank you, the American people for giving me the great honor of allowing me to serve as your President. When the Lord calls me home whenever that may be, I will leave with the greatest love for this country of ours and eternal optimism for its future.

I now begin the journey that will lead me into the sunset of my life. I know that for America there will always be a a bright dawn ahead.

Thank you my friends. May God always bless you.

Sincerely,
Ronald Reagan

tough, uncompromising and shrewd. But none of that helped him when it came to seeing his mother being devoured by an unstoppable disease.

Women, on the other hand, talk freely to me about watching a parent or even a spouse being conquered by Alzheimer's. They inhabit the experience fully, with its sorrows, its calm stretches, its dramatic explosions and even its humorous moments. If the disease is still young, they ask, "What's it like later on?" And they sincerely want to know. If they're witnessing the end stages, they can say without flinching what we all come to realize—those stages are easier. There is no fight left, no terror in the eyes, no awareness of being devoured. The person who used to be present is in a different place, far away from everything they once knew, yet seemingly content to drift there. One woman said to me, "If you think about it, they have no stress. Without memory, everything's always new."

> **66** *The disease is a vanishing into the valley of the shadow, and no one else can follow.* **99**

Maybe women are a little more willing to live alongside death and dying because, on a cellular level, we understand birth. Whether or not we end up having children, the capacity was given to us. It's encoded in our cells and our psyches. Death is, after all, just the closing of the circle. So we bend over bedsides, listen to repeated phrases and fragmented sentences—a strange kind of haiku those with Alzheimer's use. We choose when and where to shed tears, usually in private and never in front of the person who has slipped away from us. We learn to live moment to moment, because they do, and it's one way of maintaining contact.

Mostly we learn the hard lesson of acceptance. It does no good to ask why. There is no answer to that question. Asking instead, "How can I help?" ushers in only one answer: Just be there. Show up and listen, even to the silences. Deep in the silence beneath the surface of the disease is a soul that can't have Alzheimer's, a soul that still wants to be heard.

Teen Caregiver

By Lindsey Jordan,
who is 16 years old and lives in Southern California

My childhood is filled with so many wonderful family memories. My dad was a health-care professional and taught at various colleges. My mom worked part-time, and I was blessed and lucky to be a working actor and singer. My mom and dad introduced me to volunteerism when I was very young. Over the years, I learned the importance of bringing hope and happiness to others and feeling very fortunate every moment for all that I had. I learned and believed that together ordinary people could do great things.

But nothing in my life prepared me for Alzheimer's, the unforgiving and relentless disease that stole my dad's memories and robbed us of a lifetime of adventures.

Dad began showing signs of dementia in his late 40s. In 2002, when he was only 51, he was diagnosed with younger-onset Alzheimer's disease. I was 8 years old when Alzheimer's chose me to be a caregiver. (I'm 16 now.) It didn't care how old the patient or caregiver was.

Caregiving is a 24-hour-a-day job, and I helped Mom wherever I could. As a young child, I remember helping Dad get dressed, tying his shoes and preparing his breakfast, all before I went to school. I often held his hand so he wouldn't wander and get lost. I worried when he did. To calm both our fears, I often read and sang to him. All the simple things we took for granted became much more difficult.

When I was a child, Alzheimer's meant my dad was sick. Now as a young woman, my knowledge of Alzheimer's has led me to understand the harsh reality of this disease. My biggest sadness comes from knowing that this Alzheimer's has already taken my dad from me. Although I know he will always be with me in my heart, the reality is that my father will never see me reach those special milestones in my life, and I will never get to see the love and pride on Dad's face as I realize my dreams. He won't see me graduate from high school or college. He won't be by my side walking me down the aisle or smiling as his grandchildren take their first steps.

> *66 My father will never see me reach those special milestones in my life, and I'll never get to see the love and pride on Dad's face as I realize my dreams. 99*

Although I try to be strong, it has been extremely stressful and absolutely devastating to watch what this disease has done to my dad, my family and our friends. I wish no one ever has to learn firsthand what it's like to struggle financially because of this disease or shed tears of frustration and pain because they are worried about their loved ones and their own future.

As for me, I find comfort in being an Alzheimer advocate. I participate in Alzheimer's Association Memory Walk, give speeches and coordinate Alzheimer awareness events. I have had the opportunity to travel to Sacramento, California, and Washington, D.C., where I've shared my story with our elected officials and have asked for their continued support in the fight for a cure.

Sadly, my dad is in the final stages of Alzheimer's. His once warm eyes stare blankly at me now. He's unable to remember I am anyone he knows, let alone his daughter.

My dad's legacy of goodness and compassion lives within me. Although his memories are long gone, I still remember.

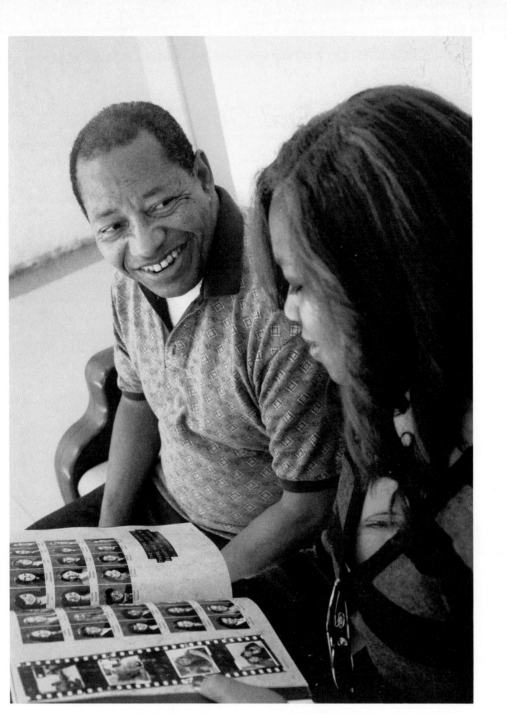
Lindsey Jordan with her dad, Charles.

"The Sad Goodbye"

*By former First Lady Laura W. Bush,
who heads the Laura Bush Foundation for America's Libraries*

*F*or years I've been an advocate for health concerns like breast cancer and heart disease because I believe lifelong good health begins with awareness. This truth has helped shape our fight against HIV/AIDS, heart disease and various cancers, but the same lesson can be applied to another leading cause of death in America: Alzheimer's disease. Today it's estimated that 5.3 million Americans are living with Alzheimer's disease, and someone develops a new case every 70 seconds. And while 11 million Americans serve as unpaid caregivers to those affected by Alzheimer's, their stories often go untold. They're on the front lines of fighting a disease that shows no reverence for a life well-lived. They see the slow fade of a once-vibrant life. Their experiences can help raise awareness and spur research to find a cure, so we can build a future in which Alzheimer's no longer exists.

In writing my memoir, *Spoken From the Heart*, I reflected on my own family's experience with Alzheimer's. What my mother noticed first was that my father could no longer fill out bank deposit slips. He would stare at the lines on the forms, a look of confusion washing over his face. So Mother began to make the deposits for him. We never got a diagnosis of Alzheimer's or a specific form of cognitive failing. But we saw his mind erode. Once, he asked our daughter Barbara to get him some "B&Bs." He meant M&Ms, but he kept saying "B&Bs." In her 10-year-old way, she understood him and came out of the grocery store with the brown bag of the bright candy just the same. When my mother took Daddy to the doctor, one of the questions on the cognition test was, "Who is the president?" And my father couldn't remember President Clinton's name. Then the doctor asked, "Who was the last president?" And Daddy had no idea, even though it was my father-in-law, George H.W. Bush.

Mother quickly learned that caring for someone suffering from Alzheimer's requires constant sacrifice. One day, my father walked in the house, set his car keys on the table and announced that he was not going to drive again. He quit forever that afternoon, and all the driving fell to my mother. For years Daddy had been the driver, taking Mother on Sunday drives to bird-watch. Now it was her responsibility. If she did not take him out, he would not leave the house. She resigned from her ladies bridge club and began to ferry my father around. She drove him to Midland's indoor mall, where they could walk undisturbed. She drove him to see his friends. But then he began to fall, and she was afraid to take him too far from home. Friends visited. They came to Daddy when he could no longer come to them. That's one of the luxuries of living a long time in a small town. Still, my parents' world shrank as Daddy became more and more housebound.

Watching Mother look after Daddy, it was clear to me that caring for a loved one suffering from Alzheimer's is a burden that cannot be carried alone. My mother was fortunate she was able to hire help. Friends and acquaintances would call with the name of someone who had assisted one of their relatives, and so she found a man to come in each morning to help Daddy bathe and dress, and she had other people who came through during the day to help.

I always felt bad that I wasn't able to pitch in more, especially in the last months of Daddy's life, because they fell during George's campaign for governor. Looking back now, I see other things I wish we had done. Daddy always loved music. He loved Glenn Miller, Glen Campbell and Jerry Jeff Walker's "London Homesick Blues." I wish we had played more music for him during those last few years. Brain researchers say that songs are imprinted in our memories longer than many other things.

It wasn't until after Daddy was gone that we realized what a weight his illness had been. About a year after Daddy died, Mother told me that she felt well again. She said she realized then how the constant vigilance of caregiving had left her feeling almost physically ill. As the burden of caring for Daddy was lifted and her own sense of well-being returned, Mother was able to focus on parts of her life that had been on hold. She began to tend to the house Daddy had built for her: reupholstering the chairs, replacing the drapes and fixing the myriad things that had gone unrepaired while Daddy was in decline.

Alzheimer's and dementia in general are often called "the long goodbye," but to me they are "the sad goodbye." So often, as with our family, we don't say goodbye when we can. We don't recognize that moment when the person we love still knows enough, still comprehends enough to hear our words and answer them. We miss that moment, and it never comes again.

I'm grateful for ongoing efforts to bring about a future in which our children and grandchildren will not have to worry about missing that moment. Without action, it's expected that Alzheimer's will claim the lives of more than 16 million Americans by 2050, and someone will develop a new case every 33 seconds—twice as often as today.

We've seen so much progress in our battle against stroke, cancer and heart disease. The same can be true for treating and curing Alzheimer's. Greater dialogue will lead to greater awareness. Purposeful investments can stimulate successful research. And together, we can help bring an end to heartbreaks caused by the sad goodbye.

Carrying My Father's Memories

By Soleil Moon Frye, who started acting at age 5 and is known worldwide as the title character in the Punky Brewster *TV series. Her documentary,* Sonny Boy, *chronicling her road trip to Iowa with her father, has won numerous film festival awards. She is an Alzheimer's Association Champion.*

My father, Virgil Frye, was an actor, an artist, a Golden Gloves boxing champion and, most proudly, a civil rights activist. He marched with Martin Luther King, and he loved to paint. He was quite a Renaissance man.

He wasn't perfect. He lived in the moment, and although he was not always there in typical father ways, he was there with love. When I was a little girl, he would dance me to sleep, and he always told the most colorful stories. At Christmastime, he would make fudge and wrap it in tinfoil for me. Looking back, that was better than any toy I could ever have received. He was eccentric and wild, but he was my dad.

It all started with the little things when he was in his early 50s, or maybe even younger— too young for us to suspect anything was wrong. He would forget where he parked his car or put his keys. He didn't know what day it was, and he would stumble over the names of the people he was with and where he was. He covered his walls with Post-it notes as everyday reminders.

We thought it was just Dad being crazy. We would tell each other half-joking, "Dad is losing his mind." We did not know that he actually was losing his mind, his memories fading off into a gray, empty space. As he drifted away a little more every day, we desperately tried to hold on to him.

We did not know the name for what was happening to him. Our family was lost and being torn apart, and my heart broke as we journeyed through the long goodbye we eventually came to know as Alzheimer's disease.

> 66 *We would tell each other half-joking, 'Dad is losing his mind.' We didn't know that he actually was losing his mind, his memories fading off into a gray, empty space.* 99

Before it was too late, I wanted to have one last chance to get to know my dad. So we drove cross-country from Los Angeles to his hometown in Iowa, retracing his history. Along the way, we had our emotional ups and downs, traveling the open road, sharing a lifetime of memories. Both of us knew that only one of us would be able to carry those memories on.

Today, my father does not speak. When I see him, he stares off, somewhere between this world and the next. Some months ago as I stood beside him, I sang him a song he used to sing to me. His eyes were closed, and a teardrop fell from the corner of his eye. I believe that whatever world he is in, he could hear me—and that even if it was only for a moment, he knew it was his little girl who has always loved him.

I sang my song for him, for us, for the memories that once were and the memories that I would carry on for him. I sang for those like him who can remember no more.

A Woman's Disease

Is There a Cure? Is There Hope?

The Rush Alzheimer's Disease Center in Chicago is one of the leading laboratories conducting Alzheimer research.

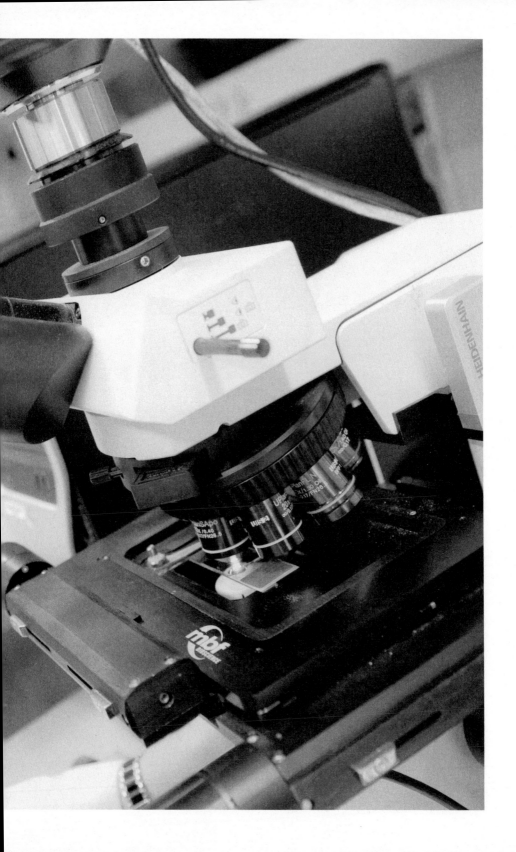

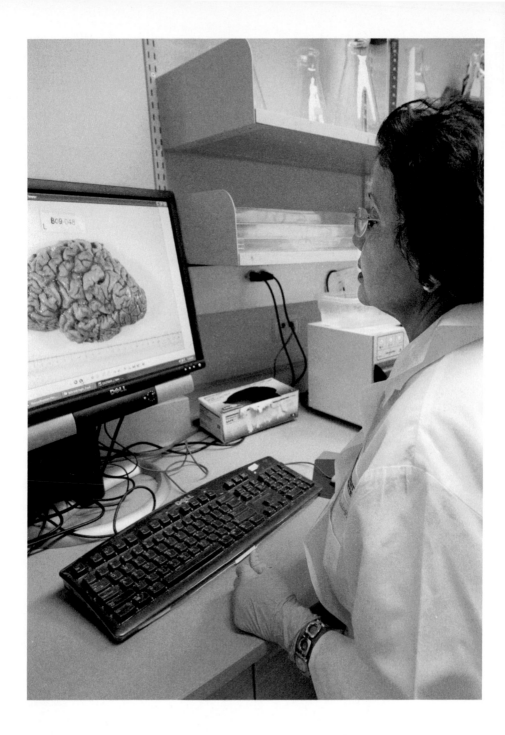

alzheimer's ९५ association®

KNOW the
10 SIGNS
EARLY DETECTION MATTERS

Memory loss that disrupts daily life may be a symptom of Alzheimer's, a fatal brain disease that causes a slow decline in memory, thinking and reasoning skills. Every individual may experience one or more of these signs in different degrees. If you notice any of them, please see a doctor. For more information, visit www.alz.org.

1. *Memory loss that disrupts daily life*

2. *Challenges in planning or solving problems*

3. *Difficulty completing familiar tasks at home, at work or at leisure*

4. *Confusion with time or place*

5. *Trouble understanding visual images and spatial relationships*

6. *New problems with words in speaking or writing*

7. *Misplacing things and losing the ability to retrace steps*

8. *Decreased or poor judgment*

9. *Withdrawal from work or social activities*

10. *Changes in mood and personality*

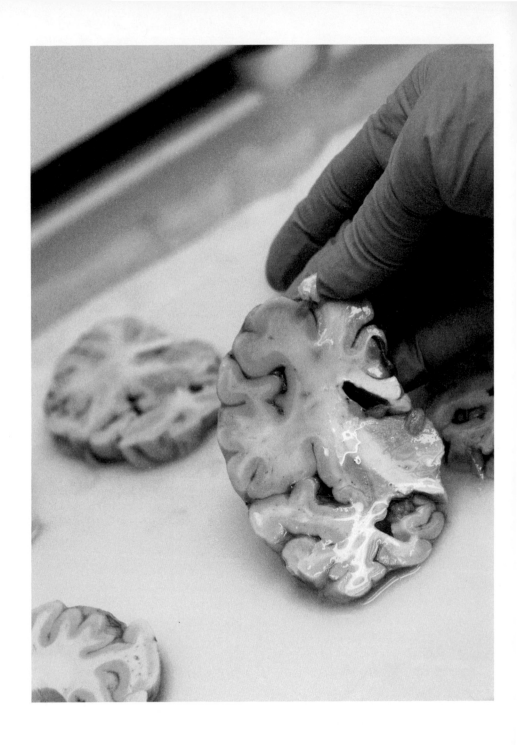

Is There a Cure? Is There Hope?

By Maria Carrillo, Ph.D.

Hope is not a dream, but a way of making dreams become reality.

—*Cardinal Leon Joseph Suenens*

Hundreds of scientists—from nonprofit groups, government, universities and drug companies—are working with unprecedented cooperation to better identify and treat Alzheimer's disease before it robs us of our memories and lives.

One of the keys may be discovering more of what are known as biomarkers—substances or molecules in the body that indicate the presence of a disease. Researchers so far have tentatively identified a number of these for Alzheimer's that suggest the disease exists as a continuum, progressing from early, detectable signs to—maybe 10 or 15 years later—full-blown Alzheimer dementia. The development of biomarker research, and our eventual ability to identify Alzheimer's years before its outward symptoms develop, may be our most promising path to preventing the disease from ever taking hold.

However—and it is a big "however"—such identification does not mean effective treatment, let alone prevention, of this complex disease is close at hand. Biomarkers remain experimental. And, in fact, without treatment options, a biomarker is just a road sign on a highway we are still learning to navigate.

So to answer succinctly the questions posed by this chapter's title:

> "Is There a Cure?" **No.**
> "Is There Hope?" **Yes.**

The truth is, we are making genuine progress in understanding this complex disease. Symptoms are being recognized earlier. Diagnoses have become highly accurate. Several drugs appear to improve thinking and memory in some people with Alzheimer's, if not yet slowing the disease's progression. As a result, indications are that we are moving closer to having the tools we need to confront the burgeoning Alzheimer epidemic.

This chapter explores all of those initiatives. It pinpoints what strategies individuals can follow as well as what studies, policies and financial support we as a society must create to propel us toward more effective therapies and, ultimately, a cure.

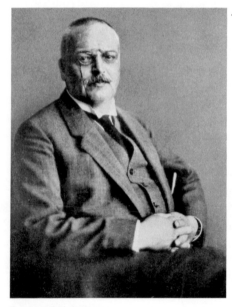
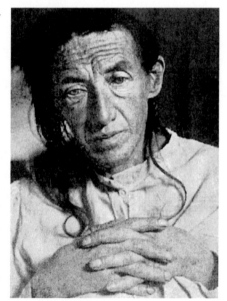

Dr. Alois Alzheimer   Frau Auguste D

The first case

A German neurologist, Dr. Alois Alzheimer, first described the disease that would come to bear his name at a scientific meeting in 1906. "Frau Auguste D" had been his patient since 1901, suffering, at age 52, from a perplexing group of behaviors that included memory loss and difficulty both speaking and understanding what was said to her. When she died, Frau Auguste D's family gave Dr. Alzheimer permission to perform an autopsy, which included a detailed study of her brain. He discovered that her brain had shrunk dramatically, and using newly developed staining techniques and a microscope, he saw unusual protein deposits called amyloid plaques and neurofibrillary tangles that are to this day the hallmark characteristics that doctors and scientists find in the brains of people with Alzheimer's disease.

From a century of further study, we today know this about Alzheimer's:

- It is a progressive, incurable and fatal disease in which cells in certain parts of the brain are destroyed, eventually leaving patients unaware of the world around them and unable to care for themselves.

- From the onset of symptoms, patients begin a relentless downward course, culminating in death usually within 2 to 15 years.

- It is not a normal part of aging, but a disease process that begins as many as 10 to 20 years before outward symptoms become apparent. This is a period in which we may be able to most effectively intervene.

The basics

Alzheimer's disease, a brain disorder that causes memory loss and other cognitive impairments, is the most common type of age-related dementia. An estimated 5.3 million Americans currently have Alzheimer's disease,[1] and this number is expected to explode to as many as 16 million people by 2050.[2] Worldwide, the numbers are as astounding: More than 35 million people were estimated to have dementia in 2009,[3] and as the world's population ages, the global prevalence of Alzheimer's disease will continue to geometrically increase.

5.3 million Americans—most of them women— currently have Alzheimer's disease.

Memory loss is usually the first symptom of Alzheimer's disease, but over time a person with the disease experiences other gradually worsening symptoms, including changes in personality, a decline in the ability to speak and understand what others say, poor decision-making ability and an inability to care for oneself. Twenty years ago, when a person or family member noticed these changes, there was little a physician could do to determine whether, in fact, the person was suffering from Alzheimer's disease or another type of dementia. Now, thanks to better tests of mental status and memory and improved imaging methods, such as those for breast cancer, colon cancer, depression, etc., experienced clinicians are routinely making Alzheimer's disease diagnoses with 90 percent accuracy.

Women and Alzheimer's

More women than men have Alzheimer's disease and other dementias, in large part because women live longer than men and the risk of developing dementia increases dramatically as a person ages. Approximately 5 percent of people between the ages of 71 and 79 have dementia, compared to more than 37 percent of those over age 90.[4] Yet while being a woman may not, in itself, increase the risk of developing Alzheimer's disease, other differences may exist between women and men with respect to the disease process, the symptoms that are observed and, possibly, the response to therapy. For example, one recent study looked at the prevalence of mild cognitive impairment (MCI), which is thought to be a precursor to Alzheimer's disease, in a group of elderly people with no dementia. This study found that the prevalence of MCI increased with age and was higher in men compared to women. The study's authors suggested that women may transition to Alzheimer dementia directly, albeit at a later age, rather than passing through the MCI phase first,[5] but more research needs to be done to clarify this issue.

> *One study showed 80 percent of women at age 90—but only 24 percent of men— had Alzheimer's.*

Studies vary with regard to whether women have a higher incidence of dementia and/or Alzheimer's disease. For example, a pooled analysis of four large population-based studies in Europe showed significant gender differences among the oldest old; among women there was a doubling of the number of new cases of Alzheimer's disease from age 85 to 90, compared to little increase among men. At 90 years of age, more than 80 percent of women, but only 24 percent of men had Alzheimer's, a finding that could be partially explained by a lower mortality rate among women in this age group, which results in a larger number surviving with the disease.[6] However, in another large study in the United States, no significant difference in dementia risk was noted between males and females.[7]

Whether or not there are differences in incidence of the disease, there are other differences between men and women with respect to their risk of developing Alzheimer's disease, the progression of the disease and its response to therapy.[8] Estrogen is the most frequently cited difference, but the many other differences between the brains of women and men may also play a role. For example, structural differences exist in how women's and men's brains are organized, and women's and men's brains also have different genetic mechanisms independent of hormone action. In addition, studies have shown that certain behaviors, such as retrieval of emotional memories, use different areas of the brain in women compared to men. There are also differences between women and men in neurotransmitter systems; and in animal studies, chronic stress causes more damage in males to the area of the brain responsible for long-term memory (the hippocampus) in comparison to females.

Diagnosing Alzheimer's disease

Recognizing warning signs and obtaining an early diagnosis offer numerous benefits to patients and families. Not only may they get treatments that could relieve some of the symptoms, people with Alzheimer's can also get access to clinical trials and community resources, such as the Alzheimer's Association, which can help individuals and families deal with the practical and emotional aspects of the diagnosis. The diagnostic process may also either uncover or rule out other conditions that can mimic some of the symptoms of Alzheimer's disease—for example, depression, stroke or a reaction to (or the interaction of) certain drugs.

There is no single, simple test that a physician can use to diagnose Alzheimer's disease. The patient's medical and family history can be quite revealing, and the clinician will likely assess memory and cognition with paper-and-pencil and verbal tests. These tests are designed to evaluate everyday mental skills such as the ability to name, remember and repeat the names of common objects, and follow simple three-part instructions. The physician will also conduct a physical and neurologic exam and take blood and urine samples to test for a wide variety of disorders such as diabetes, kidney or liver disease, and thyroid abnormalities. Finally, the standard medical workup for Alzheimer's disease today often includes an MRI scan to look for evidence of tumors, strokes or head trauma. These conditions can all produce symptoms that may be mistaken for Alzheimer's disease.

This emphasis on early diagnosis points toward a 10-to-15-year window when a person has biological changes or indicators that portend more serious events, such as the onset of symptoms of dementia. Potentially, this could present an opportunity to intervene with therapies that interrupt the progression of the earliest biological changes that may signal Alzheimer's disease. The eventual result: Alzheimer's could become a manageable disease before the onset of dementia and irreversible memory loss. An apt analogy might be how the detection of high cholesterol, not itself a debilitating condition, may allow for treatment and subsequent prevention of a heart attack.

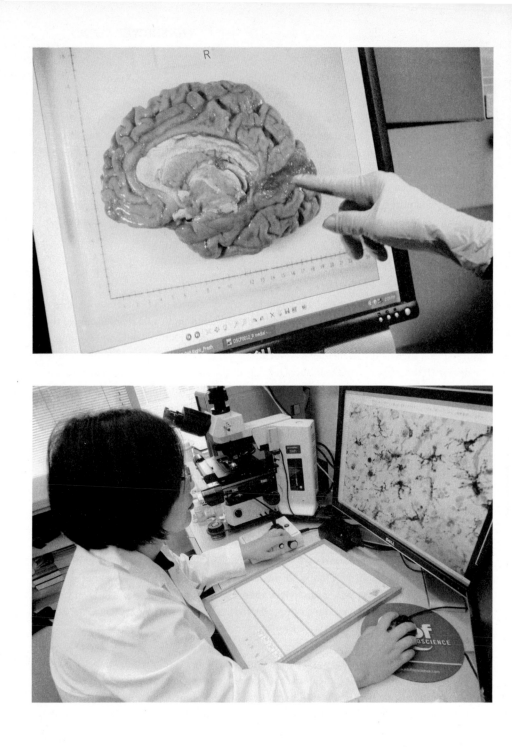

A new understanding of Alzheimer's

The current criteria for diagnosing Alzheimer's disease were established in 1984, when little was known about the genetic and molecular events that result in disease,[9] and before imaging technologies that can reveal the dysfunction or death of brain cells had become available. Developed by the National Institute of Neurological and Communicative Disorders and Stroke (NINCDS, now NINDS) and the Alzheimer's Disease and Related Disorders Association (ADRDA, now the Alzheimer's Association), these criteria required a physical evaluation as well as assessment of cognitive, emotional and brain functioning (known as neuropsychological testing) to classify patients as having probable or possible Alzheimer's disease. A definite diagnosis was made only with confirmation by a detailed study of the brain tissue at autopsy. Neuropsychological testing covered eight cognitive domains, and a diagnosis of probable Alzheimer's disease required progressive impairment in at least two of these domains. Memory is the most common of these domains to be affected; others include concentration, problem solving and language.

Biomarkers, possible indicators of the disease, offer the potential for making not only an earlier diagnosis but one that is more precise and more informative. Scientists have now identified a number of possible Alzheimer's disease biomarkers, including:

- **Biomarkers of beta-amyloid pathology.** Beta-amyloid pathology shows up as "plaques" in the brain and was first seen more than 100 years ago by Dr. Alzheimer.

- **Biomarkers of injury to brain cells (neurons).** Neuronal injury can be assessed by measuring levels in the spinal fluid of the protein "tau," which forms the tangles found in Alzheimer's-diseased brains.

- **Biomarkers of neuronal dysfunction.** Metabolic activity in different areas of the brain can indicate problems with certain brain cells and can be measured using positron emission tomography (PET) scans.

- **Biomarkers of neurodegeneration.** Assessed by using magnetic resonance imaging (MRI) scans, these biomarkers measure brain atrophy that results from the death of brain cells.

- **Genetic markers** that relate to a person's risk of developing disease or that may predict the course of disease.

This new push to find and validate biomarkers could allow doctors to make a firm diagnosis or perhaps a prediction of Alzheimer's even before symptoms are evident. In fact, scientists recently reported compelling evidence that PET scans and tests of spinal fluid can reveal some Alzheimer biomarkers before dementia symptoms arise. Biomarkers—some already discovered, others being sought—also could reveal how a treatment is working, which could open up entire new avenues leading to a possible prevention or cure.

Biomarkers could lead to making Alzheimer's a manageable disease before the onset of irreversible memory loss.

Studies such as the Alzheimer's Disease Neuroimaging Initiative (ADNI), the Australian Imaging, Biomarker, and Lifestyle Flagship Study of Ageing (AIBL) and global efforts known as World Wide ADNI, led by the Alzheimer's Association, have begun to establish biomarker profiles that appear to correlate with different stages of disease. For example, a recent study from ADNI identified an "Alzheimer's disease signature" based on measurements of beta amyloid and p-tau in the spinal fluid that appeared to predict whether a person with MCI would go on to develop Alzheimer's disease within five years.[10] Interestingly, the signature was also present in more than a third of cognitively normal subjects, suggesting that Alzheimer's disease-related changes in the brain may be detectable even before problems with memory and thinking appear.

With the identification of a number of possible biomarkers, we are coming to understand that Alzheimer's disease exists as a continuum, progressing from early, yet detectable, changes in the brain to full-blown Alzheimer dementia. Thus, in 2009, the National Institute on Aging and the Alzheimer's Association convened three workgroups to update the diagnostic criteria so that they would better reflect the full range of the disease from its earliest effects to its eventual impact on mental and physical function.

Their reports focused on three different phases of the disease:

- A pre-symptomatic, or pre-clinical, phase occurring many years before symptoms become evident.

- A symptomatic phase characterized by mild problems in the ability to think, learn and remember, enough to be noticed and measured but not enough to impair the ability to live independently or carry out everyday activities. This phase is what is currently referred to as MCI.

- Alzheimer dementia, when the disease has progressed to the point that the person has markedly impaired memory and thinking abilities and cannot function independently.

The proposed new diagnostic criteria have sparked a considerable discussion and debate. While nearly everyone agrees that the disease begins long before symptoms appear, the methods for identifying who will go on to develop the disease are still relatively new and will require many years of study before they will be universally accepted and used clinically. For now, these tools are meant to be used for research purposes only, not to diagnose people who have no symptoms. Indeed, until better treatments are available, many argue there is little reason to identify people who have no outward signs of the disease.

Predicting individual risk

Understanding risk factors for any disease, but particularly one as common and complex as Alzheimer's, is the first step toward developing new treatments and/or preventive strategies. Currently identified Alzheimer risk factors include:

Age

Age is the most important risk factor for Alzheimer's disease. Indeed, one study showed that the incidence of dementia doubles approximately every five to six years after age 65,[11] meaning that among individuals 80 to 85 years of age, as many as 40 to 45 percent have some form of dementia. Coupled with a rapidly aging worldwide population, this means the incidence of Alzheimer's is increasing astronomically.

Scientists have made great progress in understanding the fundamental molecular mechanisms underlying aging. Their research suggests not only that there are changes in the regulation of pathways involved in neurodegenerative diseases but that the rate of aging may be modifiable by targeting these pathways,[12] opening the possibility of novel ways to treat diseases like Alzheimer's. Moreover, there is a wealth of evidence suggesting that education, physical activity, overall health and genetics may affect the rate of age-related cognitive decline.

Genetics

Late-onset Alzheimer's disease (LOAD), with the onset of symptoms after age 65, is the most common form of Alzheimer's. It is not considered a genetic disease because no single gene determines if an individual will develop the illness. However, genetics undoubtedly play a role in the disease because having a first-degree relative with Alzheimer's increases the risk for getting the disease. In addition, a rare form of the disease called early-onset familial Alzheimer's disease (eFAD), which typically appears before age 50 (sometimes as early as the late 20s), is hereditary—if a parent has the disease, his or her offspring have a 50-50 chance of also being affected. Most cases of eFAD have been linked to mutations (genetic changes) in a gene called presenilin-1 (PS1); at least two other genes, PS2 and amyloid precursor protein (APP), have also been linked to eFAD. Genetic testing can be used to predict whether a person will develop eFAD; however, many people choose not to get genetic testing for a progressive, incurable and ultimately fatal disease.

Americans across the political spectrum overwhelmingly believe it's the government's responsibility to help find a cure.

Some genes also raise a person's risk of developing Alzheimer's. In 1993, a team of scientists showed that a variant in the APOE gene, called APOE-e4, confers a high risk of developing LOAD. The APOE gene produces a protein called apolipoprotein, which shuttles cholesterol, other fat-carrying proteins and other fat-soluble substances through the bloodstream. To this day, APOE-e4 remains the strongest genetic predictor of risk, although many individuals with the gene variant never get Alzheimer's disease while others who lack the variant do get the disease. Overall, a person's risk of developing LOAD increase about 12-to-15-fold if he or she has two copies of the APOE-e4 gene (one inherited from each parent). People with two copies of the APOE-e4 gene also have a much younger age of onset than those who develop Alzheimer's but have only one copy or no copies of this variant.[13]

Scientists believe that, with time, other genes will be found that influence the risk of developing Alzheimer's disease, and they are scanning and sequencing the entire genome to find genes and mutations that are associated with the disease. One such gene, identified in 2007 and called SORL1, is involved in transporting amyloid protein. Another recently identified gene is called TOMM40. This gene sits near the APOE gene and may have an even stronger relationship with age of onset than APOE variants do. TOMM40 exists as either a short, long or very long form, with long forms associated with earlier

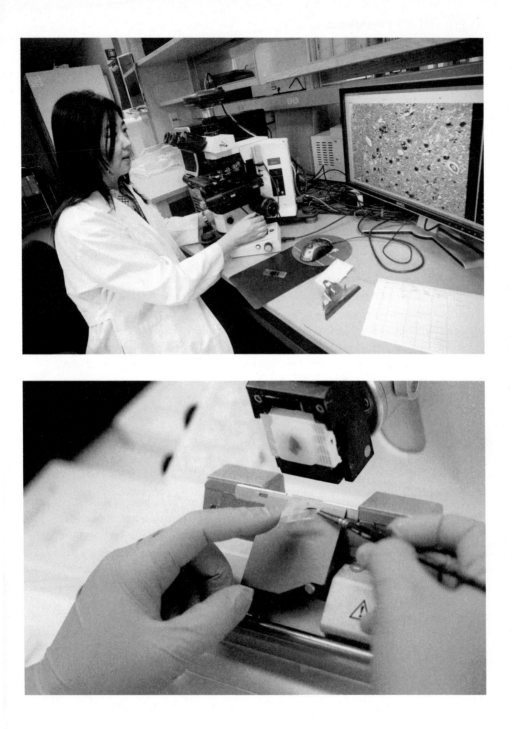

age of onset. Even more recently, variants in a gene called FTO, which is associated with obesity and diabetes, were shown to be associated with an increased risk of developing Alzheimer's disease, especially in the presence of APOE-e4.

Genetics may also play a protective role in the development of Alzheimer's. Relatives of non-demented elderly people face a risk 11 times lower than the risk for relatives of people with Alzheimer's.[14]

Diabetes/insulin resistance

As with Alzheimer's disease, the incidence of obesity, diabetes and insulin resistance is skyrocketing around the world. Many studies have shown that all of these metabolic conditions increase a person's risk of developing Alzheimer's or cognitive impairment. In one study, diabetes was shown to increase the risk of developing Alzheimer's disease by 65 percent[15]; in another study limited to older women, the risk of developing cognitive impairment doubled in women with diabetes or impaired fasting glucose, a pre-diabetic condition.[16] However, in the Framingham Study, diabetes was not shown to increase the risk of developing Alzheimer's disease.[17]

In one study of older women, those with diabetes had twice the risk of cognitive decline.

Insulin resistance refers to an inability of the cells in the body to dispose of blood sugar (glucose) through the action of insulin. This causes the pancreas to secrete more insulin, leading to a related condition, hyperinsulinemia. When the pancreas cannot keep up with the need for more insulin, a person can develop glucose intolerance, or an inability to use glucose efficiently as a body fuel. Glucose intolerance is also called "pre-diabetes," and if untreated can lead to diabetes. Obesity (referred to in the scientific literature as adiposity, or the amount of fat tissue in the body) is associated with a higher risk of insulin resistance, and there is evidence that weight loss can lower insulin resistance.

This is important with regard to Alzheimer's disease because insulin resistance and high insulin levels are associated with a higher risk of cognitive decline, particularly problems with memory. This association is even stronger in people with the APOEe4 gene variant. Insulin resistance also contributes to cardiovascular disease, which also increases the risk of Alzheimer's.

Understanding the mechanism by which insulin resistance and high insulin levels affect the brain and the development of Alzheimer's disease could lead to new treatment options and preventive strategies. One possible link is a chemical in the body called insulin degrading enzyme (IDE), which has been shown to degrade not only insulin but beta amyloid as well. Decreased function of this enzyme could theoretically increase risk of Alzheimer's disease, although this has not been proven.

Complicating the situation, while insulin has been shown to affect beta-amyloid metabolism, there is evidence that diabetes is not associated with an increased amount of plaques and tangles.[18] Nonetheless, insulin and IDE may affect cognition and the development of Alzheimer's disease independently of plaque formation. It may be that insulin resistance is related to elevated levels of chemicals called free radicals that damage the brain through a process called oxidative stress, and this may be the link to cognitive dysfunction and Alzheimer's disease. Other contributing factors may be substances produced by fatty tissue that are important in metabolism and inflammation, processes that have also been linked to brain health and cognition.

Cardiovascular disease

Obesity is a risk factor not only for diabetes, but for cardiovascular disease as well. In addition, other vascular risk factors such as hypertension, high cholesterol and atherosclerosis have been associated with both vascular dementia and Alzheimer dementia. Indeed, the link between the presence of APOE-e4 and Alzheimer's disease suggests a possible vascular-related mechanism for Alzheimer's, and coronary artery disease has been associated with plaques and tangles in brain tissue, particularly in APOE-e4 carriers.[19]

Head injury/brain injury

There appears to be a strong link between risk of Alzheimer's and serious head trauma, especially when injury involves loss of consciousness.[20] A head injury may also hasten the onset of Alzheimer symptoms in people who are already at heightened risk for the disease—for example, people who carry the APOE-e4 gene.[21]

Some research suggests that more mild head injuries, if there are many of them, may also increase risk of Alzheimer's.[22] Researchers have observed for quite some time that boxing and participating in other sports where head injuries are common may increase dementia risk, or cause it to develop sooner.[23] However, it's important to note that many people who sustain a severe head injury never develop Alzheimer's disease, and many people who get the disease never have a brain injury.[24] That is the nature of risk factors.

A link between traumatic brain injury (TBI) and Alzheimer's has generated news coverage as a result of some well-known athletes who developed Alzheimer-like disease at a relatively young age, and because of sports organizations publicly announcing the decision to examine the issue after what some consider a long period of neglect. The military has also taken an intense interest in the long-term consequences of TBI because of the high incidence of such injuries in war.

Depression

Depression has been linked to an increased risk of Alzheimer's disease. According to researchers, people with a history of depression are 2.5 times more likely to develop Alzheimer's disease than people who have never had depression, and this association appears to be independent of the incidence of vascular risk factors and stroke. Those who first develop depression before age 60 are especially vulnerable to Alzheimer's disease, with a nearly four-fold increased risk.[25] This is particularly relevant to women, who studies show experience depressions at significantly higher rates than men.

Estrogen

A link between declining estrogen levels and an increased risk of Alzheimer's disease has long been suspected. Estrogen is known to have positive effects on learning, memory and mood, and also influences development and degeneration in the brain. It is also thought to be neuroprotective, affecting several pathways that influence the survival of neurons, including energy production, inflammation and IGF-1 (insulin growth factor) signaling.[26] IGF-1 levels are increased in LOAD, and it is thought that this is important in disease development, possibly a sign that production is increased because brain cells are resistant to its effects.[27]

Because estrogen affects brain areas that are important for cognition, and because menopause is associated with sharp declines in the concentration of circulating estrogen, it was hypothesized that a decline in estrogen after menopause could be linked to cognitive decline and an increased risk of Alzheimer's disease. And indeed, early studies suggested that estrogen replacement therapy could protect against cognitive aging in women.[28]

However, the Women's Health Initiative Memory Study (WHIMS) showed that estrogen plus progestin therapy had an adverse rather than protective effect on cognition among women over 65 years old, particularly in women with lower cognitive function at the beginning of the trial.[29] This failure of estrogen therapy to improve cognition among older women led to a new idea, called the "critical period hypothesis," which holds that estrogen therapy is neuroprotective, but only if initiated during a critical time period, close to when natural or surgically induced menopause begins.[30] Many studies have supported this hypothesis,[31] and it is currently being investigated in at least two clinical trials to determine whether estrogen therapy given in midlife, shortly after menopause begins, may reduce the risk of developing dementia.[32]

Almost 90 percent of Americans who know someone with Alzheimer's are concerned that they or someone close to them will get it.

As with other studies of risk factors, knowing the mechanism behind increased or decreased risk is essential for the development of therapies. In the case of estrogen, its beneficial effects on brain aging and cognition appear to be related to interactions with neurons that respond to the acetylcholine, a chemical involved in the transmission of signals between neurons. Studies also show that the response of these "cholinergic" neurons to estrogen declines with age, which could explain why estrogen does not benefit cognition in elderly women. This suggests that it may be possible to treat post-menopausal women with a combination of a cholinergic enhancing drug and estrogen in the early stages of cognitive decline; however much more study will be needed to determine if this is, in fact, a realistic treatment strategy.[33]

Treating Alzheimer's Disease

There is no cure for Alzheimer's disease, and no treatment has been shown to slow its progression. However, there are several drugs that appear to improve thinking and memory in people with the disease; and other drugs can relieve some of the more troubling symptoms, such as depression and agitation.

The most widely used drug for treating Alzheimer's disease is Aricept (donepezil), which is one of a class of drugs called cholinesterase inhibitors. These drugs prevent the breakdown of a chemical called acetylcholine, which plays an important role in memory and other mental functions. In Alzheimer's disease, the cells that produce acetylcholine are gradually destroyed, so there is less acetylcholine available. Drugs that inhibit the breakdown of acetylcholine can only compensate for lowered levels of the chemical in the early stages of the disease before there has been massive loss of the cells that produce the chemical. Other cholinesterase inhibitors that are approved by the FDA include Razadyne (galantamine) and Exelon (rivastigmine).

The first approved cholinesterase inhibitor, Cognex (tacrine) is rarely used today because of its high incidence of adverse side effects.

Another FDA-approved therapy for Alzheimer's disease is Namenda (memantine), which works by interfering with a certain type of receptor on brain cells called NMDA receptors. By interfering with these receptors, the drug lowers the levels of a brain chemical called glutamate, which can destroy brain cells. When given to people with moderate-to-severe Alzheimer's disease, this drug can allow them to function more independently for several months longer than they might without the drug.

Future directions in treatment

Alzheimer's disease is a complex illness. While that may present a number of promising avenues for therapeutic intervention, it is unlikely that following a single path will bring us to an effective therapy or, ultimately, a cure. The hunt for new therapies is intimately tied to two paths: an effort to understand the fundamental mechanisms underlying the disease and the search for biomarkers of disease progression. In terms of mechanism, the most advanced hypothesis for many years is that beta amyloid is a major culprit in the disease; thus, drug discovery efforts have, in large part, focused either on preventing the production of beta amyloid, interfering with its formation into plaques, or increasing its degradation and clearance from the brain. These efforts have given rise to a number of drugs that have gone through several stages of clinical trials, but none has yet proven to be effective.

Another popular hypothesis positions tau as the central mediator of the disease, and has led to strategies that prevent the chemical modification of tau to its toxic form (p-tau), preventing the formation of p-tau tangles, or binding p-tau so it is not able to exert its toxic effects. Again, so far, none of these drugs have yet been shown effective. This is not to say that either of these hypotheses will not eventually yield new and effective drugs but only that they have not yet been successful.

Meanwhile, other disease pathways are being targeted by researchers and pharmaceutical companies. Many of these pathways are involved in nerve cell death or dysfunction. For example, mitochondria have also been implicated as being central to the Alzheimer's disease process.[34] Mitochondria are small structures in the cell that produce energy and play important roles in many cellular processes including cell death and the formation of synapses—the junctions between nerve cells that allow the passage of chemical and electrical signals. Mitochondria also produce substances that damage cells through a process called oxidative stress.

Q: How much progress has been made toward a cure?

Percentage indicates number of respondents that answered "**a great deal**" to the question.

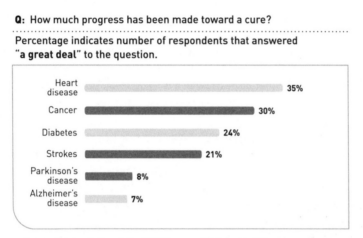

Heart disease	35%
Cancer	30%
Diabetes	24%
Strokes	21%
Parkinson's disease	8%
Alzheimer's disease	7%

Source: Alzheimer's Association 2010 Women and Alzheimer's Poll

Mitochondrial abnormalities have been seen in the brains of people with Alzheimer's, and some research suggests that targeting mitochondrial dysfunction and oxidative stress could slow or prevent the nerve damage seen in Alzheimer's disease. Other disease mechanisms that are being targeted in the search for new therapies include inflammation and insulin resistance (as discussed earlier).

Meanwhile, there is hope that non-pharmacological interventions may also be useful in the treatment of Alzheimer's disease. For example, studies of non-invasive cognitive interventions, such as training people to improve their memory or ability to recognize faces, has been shown in some studies to result in measurable changes in brain function.[35] However, much more research in this area is needed.

Clinical trials

Clinical trials are the only reliable and objective way to determine if a treatment is safe and effective. According to the National Institute on Aging, in late 2009 there were more than 90 drugs in clinical trials for Alzheimer's disease and even more awaiting approval from the FDA to enter trials.[36] There are also a large number of observational studies, which follow participants over many years to track the progression of the disease.

This large number of Alzheimer clinical studies means that large numbers of volunteers are needed, yet there are many barriers to recruiting participants for these studies. First, many people, even physicians who are treating people with Alzheimer's disease or other memory impairment, do not know the trials exist or do not know how to enroll in these trials. Many Alzheimer clinical trials also require a caregiver to participate in addition to the person with Alzheimer's, or may require travel, which further reduces the number of potential volunteers. People may be excluded for other reasons; for example, studies may exclude those with other diseases, which is a particular problem among the elderly population because older people often have multiple conditions.

To facilitate connecting more people with Alzheimer research studies, the Alzheimer's Association recently launched a free, confidential online service, Alzheimer's Association TrialMatch® (www.alz.org/trialmatch), that matches affected people, caregivers, family members, physicians and healthy volunteers with Alzheimer clinical trials that meet their criteria (e.g., diagnosis or stage of disease) and location.[37]

While the federal government will spend about $6 billion on cancer research and about $4 billion on cardiovascular disease research this coming year, it invests a fraction of that on Alzheimer research—less than $500 million a year.

While recruiting and retaining subjects remains a big roadblock to conducting clinical trials, there are other barriers as well. The trajectory of the disease presents several unique challenges. First, by the time a person has symptoms of Alzheimer's, it is likely that the disease has progressed to the point that treatments are unlikely to show significant benefit. What that means is that future trials may need to enroll people before they show outward signs of the disease. However, we now have no proven method—no biomarker—for identifying people who do not have symptoms yet are likely to go on to develop Alzheimer's.

Assuming that appropriate subjects can be identified, the next barrier is identifying relevant outcome measures. In the early or pre-symptomatic phases of the disease, changes in scores on memory or other cognitive tests may be too small to detect any improvement within a reasonable period of time. Once again, an urgent need exists for validated biomarkers that can detect a change in disease status, whether they come in the form of more sensitive cognitive tests, imaging studies or analyses of blood or spinal fluid.

Prevention

Many people believe that prevention is the only way to stop the disease from overwhelming our public health system and national economy. The good news is that there is reason to believe that Alzheimer's disease can be prevented, or at least slowed considerably, in the future.

The Nun Study is a long-term study of aging that began in 1986, enrolling 678 members of the School Sisters of Notre Dame between the ages of 75 and 102.[38] Each of the participants agreed that when they died, they would donate their brains for research. These studies confirm what others had previously noted, that the brains of some people who appear cognitively normal are, in fact, riddled with the same plaques and tangles seen in those with severe Alzheimer dementia. That raises two big questions: How is cognitive loss is averted in these people? Can we learn from them how their brain functions well even in the presence of degeneration and cell death?

Research suggests that there may be two components at work here. Brain reserve refers to differences in the brain itself that confer protection against the development of disease, while cognitive reserve refers to differences in how people use their brains to accomplish various tasks. Importantly, life experiences such as education, occupation, social interactions and leisure activities appear to increase a person's cognitive reserve, such that he or she is better able to tolerate brain damage or brain disease. In the Nun Study, for example, researchers have demonstrated a correlation between linguistic ability (i.e., the expression of complex ideas) in early life and protection against cognitive problems in late life, even in the presence of disease.[39] Other studies have demonstrated that the risk of Alzheimer's disease is associated with lifestyle factors that are potentially modifiable, including education, occupation, cognitive and leisure activities, exercise and diet.[40]

Some evidence exists that these lifestyle changes affect not only cognitive reserve but brain reserve as well by causing biological changes in the brain. For instance, in animal studies, enriching the environment—such as providing mice with a more natural living environment, stimulating activities and plenty of exercise—has been shown to modulate brain reserve by preventing or slowing the accumulation of plaques and tangles in the brain.[41] Some animal studies show other brain changes in response to exercise, including a reduction in inflammation and an elevation in factors that stimulate new brain cell growth.[42]

Thus, it appears that several strategies could help prevent Alzheimer dementia,[43] although the evidence is not conclusive.

Conclusion

Despite the current lack of effective treatments for Alzheimer's disease, progress in understanding the disease and new technologies for tracking the progression of disease suggest that we may soon have better tools to confront the oncoming public health tsunami that is Alzheimer's disease.

One of the things necessary to move research forward is a Framingham-type study for Alzheimer's disease—that is, a large, long-term study that tracks the development of cognitive impairment and Alzheimer's disease in a population of adults beginning in mid-life and throughout old age, preferably over several generations. Participants in this study would submit to repeated clinical, neuropsychological and imaging studies over their lifetimes. Data would also be collected about environmental and lifestyle factors that might influence the development of dementia. Over time, and in combination with other long-term studies such as ADNI, researchers would be able to develop something akin to the pediatric growth chart that parents of small children are familiar with, in which norms are set for various body measurements so that clinicians can be alerted when a child is not growing as expected. The adult neurological function and behavioral health chart would be designed to identify people who show early signs of cognitive, emotional, sensory and motor dysfunction.

Steps are already being taken to lay the groundwork for a study of this type. In 2006, the National Institutes of Health launched the NIH Toolbox Initiative, which seeks to assemble brief, comprehensive and well-validated assessment tools that can be used in a variety of clinical and research settings. By using common tools provided in the toolbox, clinical and research data from different groups can be compared across studies.

The Alzheimer research community has already demonstrated a commitment to collaboration that is both unprecedented and absolutely essential for addressing a problem as enormous as Alzheimer's disease. Whereas some scientists have been accustomed to protecting their data so that they are not "scooped" by someone else, Alzheimer researchers involved in large studies such as ADNI share data freely, making it easily accessible and available to other investigators around the world. The results have been remarkable—nearly every week a new important study about Alzheimer's is reported.

The problem we face is in no small part a financial one, and thus ultimately one of public policy. More research dollars are drastically needed and conducting clinical trials is enormously expensive.

Solving the Alzheimer crisis requires addressing the chronic underinvestment in Alzheimer's disease research. Only through such research will better treatments—and eventually a cure—be found. Government must take a leadership role in investing in Alzheimer research at a level that matches its impact on our economy and society—it must demonstrate the commitment to fighting Alzheimer's disease through research, education and care.

At a time of worldwide financial turmoil, both the public and private sectors need to find a way to address this problem before it overwhelms us.

ENDNOTES

1   *Alzheimer's Association, 2010 Alzheimer's Disease Facts and Figures, Alzheimer's & Dementia,* Volume 6.

2   L.E. Hebert, P.A. Scherr, J.L. Bienias, D.A. Bennett, D.A. Evens, "Alzheimer disease in the US population: prevalence estimates using the 2000 census," *Archives of Neurology,* 2003 Aug;60(8):1119-22.

3   *2009 World Alzheimer Report,* Alzheimer's Disease International.

4   B.L. Plassman, K.M. Langa, G.G. Fisher, S.G. Heeringa, D.R. Weir, M.B. Ofstedal, J.R. Burke, M.D. Hurd, G.G. Potter, W.L. Rodgers, D.C. Steffens, R.J. Willis, R.B. Wallace, "Prevalence of dementia in the United States: the aging, demographics, and memory study," *Neuroepidemiology.* 2007;29(1-2):125-32. Epub 2007 Oct 29.

5   R.C. Petersen, R.O. Oberts, D.S. Knopman, Y.E. Geda, R.H. Cha, V.S. Pankratz, B.F. Boeve, E.G. Tangalos, R.J. Ivnik, W.A. Rocca, "Prevalence of mild cognitive impairment is higher in men: The Mayo Clinic Study of Aging," *Neurology.* 2010;75:889-897.

6   K. Andersen, L.J. Launer, M.E. Dewey, L. Letenneur, A. Ott, J.R. Copeland, J.F. Dartigues, P. Kragh-Sorensen, M. Baldereschi, C. Brayne, A. Lobo, J.M. Martinez-Lage, T. Stijnen, A. Hofman. "Gender differences in the incidence of AD and vascular dementia: The EURODEM Studies," EURODEM Incidence Research Group, *Neurology.* 1999 Dec 10;53(9):1992-7.

7   B.L. Plassman, K.M. Langa, G.G. Fisher, S.G. Heeringa, D.R. Weir, M.B. Ofstedal, J.R. Burke, M.D. Hurd, G.G. Potter, W.L. Rodgers, D.C. Steffens, R.J. Willis, R.B. Wallace, "Prevalence of dementia in the United States: the aging, demographics, and memory study," *Neuroepidemiology.* 2007;29(1-2):125-32. Epub 2007 Oct 29.

8   L. Cahill, "Why sex matters for neuroscience," *Nature Reviews Neuroscience,* 2006 Jun;7(6):477-84.

9   G. McKhann , D. Drachman, M. Folstein, R. Katzman, D. Price, E.M. Stadlan, "Clinical diagnosis of Alzheimer's disease: report of the NINCDS-ADRDA Work Group under the auspices of Department of Health and Human Services Task Force on Alzheimer's Disease," *Neurology,* 1984 Jul;34(7):939-44.

10 G. De Meyer, F. Shapiro, H. Vanderstichele, E. Vanmechelen , S. Engelborghs, P.P. De Deyn, E. Coart, O. Hansson, L. Minthon, H. Zetterberg, K. Blennow , L. Shaw, J.Q. Trojanowski, for the Alzheimer's Disease Neuroimaging Initiative. "Diagnosis-Independent Alzheimer Disease Biomarker Signature in Cognitively Normal Elderly People." *Archives of Neurology*, 2010 Aug;67(8):949-956.

11 K. Ziegler-Graham, R. Brookmeyer, E. Johnson, H.M. Arrighi, 2008, "Worldwide variation in the doubling time of Alzheimer's disease incidence rates," *Alzheimer's and Dementia* 4(2008): 316-323.

12 N.A. Bishop, T. Lu, B.A. Yankner, "Neural mechanisms of ageing and cognitive decline." *Nature*, 2010 Mar 25;464(7288):529-35.

13 D. Blacker, J.L. Haines, L. Rodes, H. Terwedow, R.C. Go, L.E. Harrell, R.T. Perry, S.S. Bassett, G. Chase, D. Meyers, M.S. Albert, R. Tanzi, "ApoE-4 and age at onset of Alzheimer's disease: the NIMH genetics initiative," *Neurology*, 1997 Jan;48(1):139-47.

14 H. Payami, K. Montee, J. Kaye, "Evidence for familial factors that protect *against* dementia and out-weigh the effect of increasing age," *American Journal of Human Genetics*, 1994 Apr;54(4):650-7.

15 Z. Arvanitakis, R.S. Wilson, J.L. Bienias, D.A. Evans, D.A. Bennett, "Diabetes mellitus and risk of Al-zheimer disease and decline in cognitive function," *Archives of Neurology,* 2004 May;61(5):661-6.

16 K. Yaffe, T. Blackwell, A.M. Kanaya, N. Davidowitz, E. Barrett-Connor, K. Krueger, "Diabetes, impaired fasting glucose, and development of cognitive impairment in older women," *Neurology,* 2004 Aug 24;63(4):658-63.

17 A. Akomolafe, A. Beiser, J.B. Meigs, R. Au, R.C. Green, L.A. Farrer, P.A. Wolf, S. Seshadri, "Diabetes mellitus and risk of developing Alzheimer disease: results from the Framingham Study," *Archives of Neurology,* 2006 Nov;63(11):1551-5.

18 I. Alafuzoff, L. Aho, S. Helisalmi, A. Mannermaa, H. Soininen, "Beta-amyloid deposition in brains of subjects with diabetes." *Neuropathology and Applied Neurobiology,* 2009 Feb;35(1):60-8. Epub 2008 Mar 10.

19 M.S. Beeri, M. Rapp, J.M. Silverman, J. Schmeidler, H.T. Grossman, J.T. Fallon, D.P. Purohit, D.P. Perl, A. Siddiqui, G. Lesser, C. Rosendorff, V. Haroutunian, "Coronary artery disease is associated with Alzheimer disease neuropathology in APOE4 carriers," *Neurology.* 2006 May 9;66(9):1399-404.

20 "Head trauma," Alzheimer's Association website, www.alz.org/research/science/alzheimers_preven-tion_and_risk.asp#injury, accessed 10-6-10.

21 "Can a head injury cause or hasten Alzheimer's disease or other types of dementia?" Mayo Clinic web-site, www.mayoclinic.com/health/alzheimers-disease/AN01710, accessed 10-6-10.

22 "Special Report: Researchers Find Definitive Proof that Repetitive Head Injury Accelerates the Pace of Alzheimer's Disease," Centre for Neuro Skills website, www.neuroskills.com/pr-alztbi.shtml, accessed 10-6-10. References a report published in *The Journal of Neuroscience.*

23 "Head Injuries And Alzheimer's," the Tangled Neuron website, www.tangledneuron.info/the_tangled_neuron/2007/03/head_injuries_a.html, accessed 10-6-10. References a report from *Neurosurgery.*

24 "Can a head injury cause or hasten Alzheimer's disease or other types of dementia?" Mayo Clinic web-site, www.mayoclinic.com/health/alzheimers-disease/AN01710, accessed 10-6-10.

25 M.I. Geerlings, T. den Heijer, P.J. Koudstaal, A. Hofman, M.M. Breteler, "History of depression, depres-sive symptoms, and medial temporal lobe atrophy and the risk of Alzheimer disease," *Neurology.* 2008 Apr 8;70(15):1258-64.

26 S.C. Correia, R.X. Santos, S. Cardoso, C. Carvalho, M.S. Santos, C.R. Oliveira, P.I. Moreira, "Effects of estrogen in the brain: is it a neuroprotective agent in Alzheimer's disease?" *Current Aging Science,* 2010 Jul 1;3(2):113-26.

27 E.R. Vardy, P.J. Rice, P.C. Bowie, J.D. Holmes, P.J. Grant, N.M. Hooper, "Increased circulating insulin-like growth factor-1 in late-onset Alzheimer's disease," *Journal of Alzheimer's Disease,* 2007 Dec;12(4):285-90.

28 B.B. Sherwin, "Estrogen and cognitive functioning in women," *Endocrine Reviews,* 2003 Apr;24(2):133-51.

29 M.A. Espeland, S.R. Rapp, S.A. Shumaker, R. Brunner, J.E. Manson, B.B. Sherwin, J. Hsia, K.L. Margolis, P.E. Hogan, R. Wallace, M. Dailey, R. Freeman, J. Hays, Women's Health Initiative Memory Study, "Conjugated equine estrogens and global cognitive function in postmenopausal women: Women's Health Initiative Memory Study," *Journal of the American Medical Association,* 2004 Jun 23;291(24):2959-68.

30 B.B. Sherwin, "The critical period hypothesis: can it explain discrepancies in the oestrogen-cognition literature?" *Journal of Neuroendocrinology,* 2007 Feb;19(2):77-81.

31 J.M. Daniel, J. Bohacek. "The critical period hypothesis of estrogen effects on cognition: Insights from basic research," *Biochimica et Biophysica Acta,* 2010 Jan 25. [Epub ahead of print]

32 W.W. Henderson, R.D. Brinton, "Menopause and mitochondria: windows into estrogen effects on Alzheimer's disease risk and therapy," *Progress in Brain Research,* 2010;182:77-96.

33 R.B. Gibbs, "Estrogen therapy and cognition: a review of the cholinergic hypothesis," *Endocrine Reviews,* 2010 Apr;31(2):224-53. Epub 2009 Dec 17.

34 W.E. Müller, A. Eckert, C. Kurz, G.P. Eckert, K. Leuner, "Mitochondrial dysfunction: common final pathway in brain aging and Alzheimer's disease--therapeutic aspects," *Molecular Neurobiology.* 2010 Jun;41(2-3):159-71. Epub 2010 May 12.

35 J. van Paasschen, L. Clare, R.T.Woods, D.E. Linden, "Can we change brain functioning with cognition-focused interventions in Alzheimer's disease? The role of functional neuroimaging," *Restorative Neurology and Neuroscience,* 2009;27(5):473-91.

36 National Institute on Aging Fact Sheet: Participating in Alzheimer's Disease clinical trials and studies. September 2009. NIH Publication No. 09-7484.

37 www.alz.org/research/clinical_trials/find_clinical_trials_trialmatch.asp#matchbox

38 D.A. Snowdon, "Aging and Alzheimer's disease: lessons from the Nun Study," *Gerontologist.* 1997 Apr;37(2):150-6.

39 D. Iacono, W.R. Markesbery, M. Gross, O. Pletnikova, G. Rudow, P. Zandi, J.C. Troncoso, "The Nun study: clinically silent AD, neuronal hypertrophy, and linguistic skills in early life," *Neurology.* 2009 Sep 1;73(9):665-73. Epub 2009 Jul 8.

40 M.K. Jedrziewski, V.M. Lee, J.Q. Trojanowski. "Lowering the risk of Alzheimer's disease: evidence-based practices emerge from new research," *Alzheimer's & Dementia.* 2005 Oct;1(2):152-60.

41 O. Lazarov, J. Robinson , Y.P. Tang, I.S. Hairston, Z. Korade-Mirnics, V.M. Lee, L.B. Hersh, R.M. Sapolsky, K. Mirnics, S.S. Sisodia, "Environmental enrichment reduces Abeta levels and amyloid deposition in transgenic mice," *Cell.* 2005 Mar 11;120(5):701-13.

42 C.W. Cotman, N.C. Berchtold, L.A. Christie, "Exercise builds brain health: key roles of growth factor cascades and inflammation," *Trends in Neuroscience.* 2007 Sep;30(9):464-72. Epub 2007 Aug 31.

43 L.E. Middleton, K. Yaffe, "Promising strategies for the prevention of dementia," *Archives of Neurology,* 2009 Oct;66(10):1210-5.

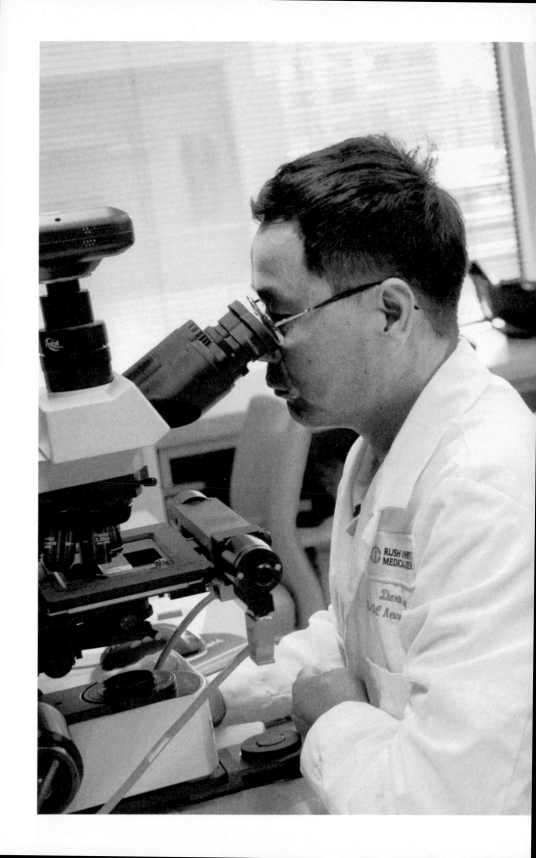

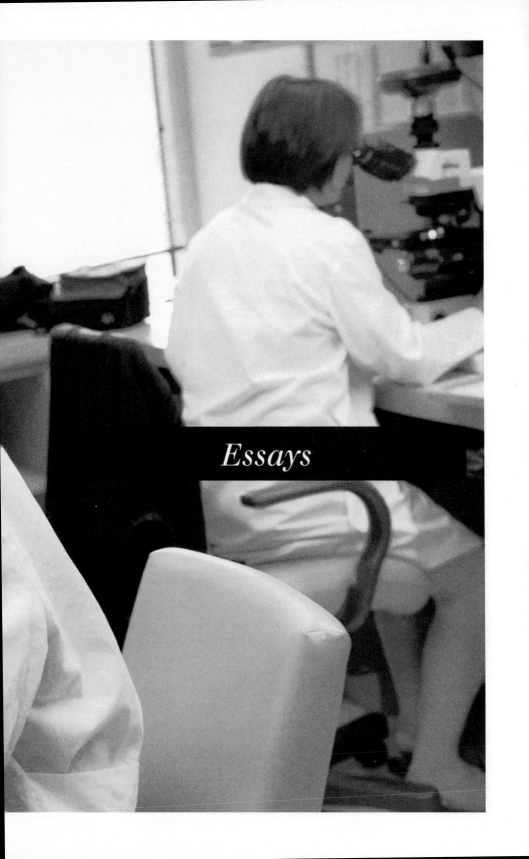

Essays

Dr. Oz's Tips for Brain Health

By Dr. Mehmet Oz, a cardiothoracic surgeon and professor of surgery at Columbia University who hosts The Dr. Oz Show, *writes a nationally syndicated column and has authored six bestselling books on health and wellness.*

As you're learning in this report, the prevalence of Alzheimer's disease is on the rise. Fortunately, with the recent Alzheimer's Disease Neuroimaging Initiative, research labs are now collaborating—instead of competing—in an innovative effort to rapidly advance our knowledge of what causes the disease and to find prevention strategies that work.

While we wait for more proof of potential Alzheimer prevention strategies, there are many good studies showing that certain lifestyle choices are associated with increasing brain health and potentially decreasing one's risk of developing Alzheimer's. And these same lifestyle choices have been proven to lower the risk of other diseases as well. So, with many health benefits—and the potential for brain protection—here are my must-follow lifestyle tips for Alzheimer prevention.

Some of the strong brain-health research, including a recent study out of Boston University, links a healthy heart with a healthy brain. Conditions such as high blood pressure, heart disease, high cholesterol and diabetes that damage heart and blood vessels are associated with increased risk of Alzheimer's and other types of dementia. Basically, your blood feeds your brain, so if your arteries are blocked, fewer nutrients get to the brain, which may lead to cognitive decline.

TIP #1: Exercise—particularly exercise that's good for the heart—may improve cognitive function. Even better? Try exercises that engage your brain as well, like a game of tennis or a yoga class. Tennis will challenge your mind to make spur-of-the-moment decisions that can strengthen cognitive function, and yoga will relieve stress and relax the brain.

TIP #2: As you probably can guess, go for a healthy diet, but there's a twist. Specific foods may reduce your risk for developing Alzheimer's when they're eaten in combination even more than when you eat them alone. A study published recently in *Archives of*

Neurology showed that a diet rich in salad dressing, nuts, fish, tomatoes, poultry, cruciferous vegetables, fruits and dark leafy greens—in combination with low intake of high-fat foods such as red meat, organ meat and butter—had a 30 percent reduced risk of Alzheimer's. These foods are all rich in folate, vitamin E and omega-3s, which suggests that these nutrients might help protect the brain from neurodegeneration. While the mechanism by which they work is still unclear, these nutrients are healthy on so many levels that you might as well load up. The next time you make dinner, try a salad of spinach, salmon and almonds to get all three of these beneficial nutrients in one meal.

TIP #3: A number of studies show that maintaining strong social interactions and engaging in regular mental activity is associated with decreased risk of cognitive decline. So my last piece of advice is to surround yourself with loved ones. Schedule that coffee date or invite your friend over for lunch. In addition, make sure you do something to challenge your mind every day, whether it's a crossword or a good book—and particularly something that is new to you. Even better, combine the two. Engage yourself in family activities that force quick decisions—like table tennis or timed board games— and you'll get your social interaction and mind challenge in one fell swoop.

Unfortunately, despite all efforts, even the healthiest person may still experience cognitive decline with age. Alzheimer's disease results from a complex interaction of factors: genetics, age, environment, lifestyle and existing medical conditions. While some of these factors can be addressed, others, such as genetics and age, are unavoidable. There are five drugs to date that have been approved by the U.S. Food and Drug Administration to address Alzheimer symptoms. On average, these drugs improve symptoms for up to 12 months in about half the individuals who take them. Moreover, a number of experimental therapies designed to go beyond treating symptoms to actually slowing or stopping the progression of Alzheimer's are in the works.

We still have a ways to go before we fully understand the causes of Alzheimer's, but new research looks promising. In the meantime, my best advice is to maintain your overall health—physical, nutritional and psychological. Exercise to improve cardiovascular health, load up your diet with fruits and vegetables rich in potent nutrients such as folate and omega-3s, and engage your mind. A healthy body could be the key to keeping your mind sharp well into old age.

Slowing Alzheimer's Down

*By Mimi Steffen, a retired schoolteacher living in Honesdale, Pennsylvania.
She is active in her local historical society, in an agency for
victims of domestic violence and in the Alzheimer's Association.*

Four years ago, at the age of 78, I was diagnosed with early-stage Alzheimer's disease. A death sentence? Eventually, yes. But not today or tomorrow. So once I got my breath back, I set my mind on two goals. One, I wouldn't keep it a secret. And two, I would continue to live life to the fullest. I'm proud to say I'm accomplishing both.

How has Alzheimer's impacted my life? As of now, there have been only some slight downsides. Of course, I don't trust my memory and must check the calendar often. Recently names have also been somewhat of a problem. But one of the benefits of everyone knowing I have Alzheimer's is that when I can't come up with a name, someone always jumps in to supply it.

> **" I was diagnosed with early-stage
> Alzheimer's. A death sentence? Eventually,
> yes. But not today or tomorrow. "**

My social life has changed some. I used to enjoy book clubs. I still love to read, but now I find that because of my short-term memory deficit, I can't participate in discussions about specific characters or incidents in a book I finished more than a few days before. I've also become aware that noisy groups bother me, so though I still love to go out, I do avoid noisy situations.

How has Alzheimer's affected my overall health? Believe it or not, I'm healthier and more cognizant of my health now than I was before my Alzheimer diagnosis. Because of a coexisting neurological condition, myasthenia gravis, my energy level and muscle strength had been gradually deteriorating. I was so wobbly walking, I needed a cane. A new neurologist ordered physical therapy. A year later, the cane is long since gone. I can do a mile on the treadmill with the elevation 7 to 9 degrees. My doctor is amazed. I believe the exercise has got to slow the dementia down.

I'm diligent about reading up on my disease and listening to the experts' recommendations. That's helped me formulate what I call my my "Best Practices" list:

1. Take all medication as directed. I take medicines for Alzheimer's, myasthenia and high blood pressure.

2. Get vigorous physical exercise. Doctors say what's good for the heart is good for the head. My internist says that the improvement he's seen in my heart condition is far greater than what could be expected from the medication alone.

3. Get vigorous mental exercise. I read a great deal, and my retention has improved, too. It used to be that it would take me all the way to the climax of a novel to realize I knew what was coming next, because I'd already read the book. Now I realize within the first page or so if I've read it already. I also enjoy doing lots of puzzles and Sudoku, and I write a quarterly column for my county Historical Society newsletter.

4. Eat a Mediterranean diet with plenty of fruits, vegetables, fish and healthy oils. In addition, I take antioxidants and Omega-3. My blood work is so much better than it was four years ago.

5. Be sure to socialize. As we get older, it seems our group of friends tends to shrink. I'm aware of this and deliberately call people for dinner or other events.

I must be conservative about how I spend my money, so it will carry me through the time when I have to go into a facility. I've already found an assisted living residence where I'll go when that day comes.

In the meantime, I've become active in the Alzheimer's Association, which includes serving on the Early Stage Advisory Group of the national organization. I'm also working as a peer volunteer in the message board community at the Alzheimer's Association website, www.alz.org.

Far from being depressed, I'm pretty optimistic. I feel that at the age of 82, I have a mission in life: to make people aware that with an early Alzheimer diagnosis and vigorous effort, the length of the downward slide can be significantly increased.

A Medical Marathon

By Eugene Fields, whose career in Ohio includes 25 years in real estate investment and management. He has successfully completed 50 marathons.

I used to think I knew what there was to know about Alzheimer's disease: memory loss. But even if I knew it all, nothing could have prepared me for what I've learned about Alzheimer's from the inside. My wife Carol's personality has changed totally. Over time, her pride and dignity have been stripped away, her self-esteem has dissipated, her anxiety has created turmoil in her mind. How could I possibly have known about the magnitude of the emotional, personal and financial devastation Alzheimer families deal with every day? And the only solution we have is to hold on to hope and believe that tomorrow will be a better day.

Carol is 72 now; we've been married for 46 wonderful years and have four children. My wife is a very spiritual person, and I'm convinced that the spirituality she cultivated within herself before she developed the disease is what helped preserve her generally calm and pleasant demeanor for so long, which I know makes her rare among people with Alzheimer's.

> **Some family members avoided being around us, as if Alzheimer's were contagious, or maybe it was just too difficult for them to see her that way.**

Carol was first diagnosed by a neurologist in November 2006. In deep denial, I sought a second opinion at the Mayo Clinic in Jacksonville, Florida, where they did lab work, a CT scan and an EEG. She saw a psychologist, a neurologist and other specialists. They said they saw possible seizure activity in her brain's temporal lobe. And on January 15, 2007, they also confirmed the diagnosis: Alzheimer's disease.

Initially, some family members avoided being around us, as if Alzheimer's were contagious, or maybe it was just too difficult for them to see her that way. For us, we focused on dealing with the disease.

The Mayo team decided not to prescribe the common Alzheimer drug Aricept because seizures can be a side effect. They did start her on an anti-seizure medication, Lamictal, and then a few months later, they added the Alzheimer medication Namenda.

Carol did extremely well on these two drugs. Her memory and alertness seemed better. She had good days and not-so-good-days, but there was no further deterioration for a while.

But about a year later, I noticed her memory worsening, and nightmares and hallucinations beginning. She thought she saw people in our house. She didn't know where she was. The doctors switched her to Aricept plus Namenda, and that worked for a few weeks. Then the hallucinations started again, worse than before.

For about a year now, it has gotten steadily worse. On bad days, Carol forgets who I am. In the mornings, she thinks I'm her deceased father, Richard. She confuses our daughter, Sharyl, with our niece, Robin. She often talks of going home when she's at home—or going to work, though she hasn't worked for five years.

She has also become fascinated with "the lady in the mirror." At first, she didn't recognize this lady as her own reflection. It scared her that "the lady" was mocking her by following her around and imitating everything she did. More recently, she sees this lady as a friend, holding conversations with her, sometimes all day long.

> 66 *When Alzheimer's first invaded our lives, we were so thankful that we had three sources of medical insurance. Now our whole financial world is in ruins, and it's down to just Medicare.* 99

For a while now, Carol has been getting up before me and waiting at the foot of the bed until I wake, when she asks me if it's OK to use the bathroom. I get up and assist her. I also now have to remind her to perform routine functions like brushing her teeth and taking a shower. And of course, I've become like a pharmacist, dispensing the scheduled medications.

It's not just the physical and emotional effects of the disease that take their toll. The dollar cost of 24-hour care is beyond belief. When Alzheimer's first invaded our lives, we were so thankful that we had three sources of medical insurance. But last year, the first one was cancelled because the benefit plan changed. A few months later, the second one, the disability coverage, ran out. And this year, the third one, our long-term care insurance, was also cancelled. Now our whole financial world is in ruins, and it's down to just Medicare. I just have to believe that the power of positive thinking and the force of the spirit will see Carol and me through.

> 66 *How could I possibly have known about the magnitude of the emotional, personal and financial devastation Alzheimer families deal with every day?* 99

Another huge challenge is caregiver stress. In order to cope, I've turned to what I've learned from my training for marathon races. First, you make it real in your mind that you're going to race 26.2 miles and accept all the challenges that will come with that. In the same way, I make it real in my mind that we are in this Alzheimer thing for the long haul. Whatever challenges will come with that, I know we'll have the inner strength to meet them.

In running, the day-in, day-out training forms a body-mind connection that teaches us to take it one mile at a time. I'm using the same technique to cope with the stresses associated with caregiving. Caregiving is also like running a hard, uphill-downhill 26.2-mile marathon, one mile at a time. You just keep putting one foot in front of the other, until you're done. So far, it's been working.

Now Carol and I are approaching the 26-mile mark, and we still take it one step at a time, one mile at a time, one day at a time. My training has taught me that focus and determination are the key and also the reward. For above all, I clearly see that emotional challenges like ours help us to seek and reach our highest good—learning, growing, supporting, giving, loving and accepting whatever comes.

Just like we have for 46 years, Carol and I are running this marathon together. With faith and assurance, we're pressing on to the finish line.

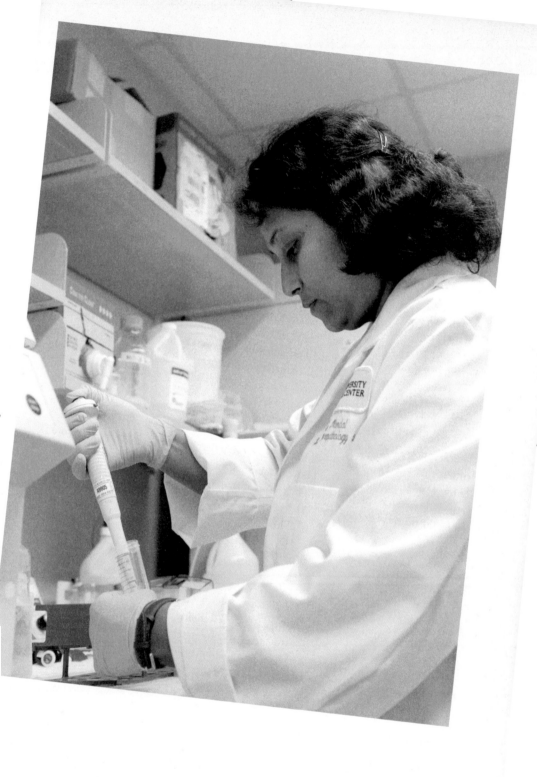

Really Early Onset

By Kris Bakowski, who is retired from a career in special events planning and marketing and lives in Athens, Georgia.

Our lives are shaped by defining moments. One of my defining moments came at the age of 46.

I had it all: a loving family, a great network of friends and a successful career. So you can imagine my shock when the neurologist told me I had "probable Alzheimer's disease." That was a defining moment that changed my life forever. The fact is, what he said made sense. I'd been having serious lapses in memory, concentration and judgment. After eight months of medical testing, Alzheimer's was confirmed. That was eight years ago.

I was scared. Not scared for me, but for my family. I've always been the one to care for them, but now I have the easy part. It's they who have to live with the hard part. The truth is that I carry a huge amount of guilt knowing my family is going to have to care for me. My son and his wife are just starting their careers, and my husband is finally settled into retirement. I'm becoming a burden right at a time when we all should be enjoying the prime of our lives. I don't want them to miss out on life because of me.

> 66 *Each time there's a wedding, anniversary, birth or graduation to celebrate, I think, 'Is this the last one I'll remember?'* 99

I worry about what's coming. Each time there's a wedding, anniversary, birth or graduation to celebrate, I think, "Is this the last one I'll remember?" My family worries about it, too. Shortly after my diagnosis, my son Alan wrote me a letter. He said, "What makes me sad is that although I will always love you, in time you won't be able to remember that I do. So I'll say it as often as I can now: I love you."

Another defining moment came when I realized that Alzheimer's is incredibly misunderstood. Many people in my life didn't want to believe that I—a so-called "normal" person they knew—had Alzheimer's, because that meant that anyone, even they, could get the disease, too. So many of them didn't want to associate with me anymore. They looked at me as if I had been struck stupid, as if I could no longer speak or think. They distanced themselves from me and my family, and that hurt. In this respect, Alzheimer's truly is a silent disease. It's silent in the sense that no one wants to talk about it.

66 *I like to think I'm living with Alzheimer's —* *rather than dying from it.* 99

So I joined with the Alzheimer's Association as an advocate to try to help remove the stigma from the disease and make Alzheimer's a public health priority. I started speaking with local groups, then state groups and then nationally. I write about it on my blog (www.creatingmemories.blogspot.com) so my friends and family can understand what this dreaded disease is all about. I can't sit idly by and do nothing, as long as I still have a voice. And I still do have my voice.

Today, at age 54 and retired on disability, I try to live as normal a life as I can, although the meaning of "normal" changes frequently.

For now, I like to think I'm living with Alzheimer's—rather than dying from it.

A Doctor's View

By Laurel Coleman, M.D.,
geriatric physician and national board member of the Alzheimer's Association

*I*t isn't supposed to be like this," Patty said. She was 67 years old and had been looking forward to retirement with her husband—traveling, visiting their children and finally enjoying more leisure time. Instead, his Alzheimer's disease is now so advanced that she cannot leave him alone, even for a minute. Like many women, Patty had spent most of her life as a caregiver for her family, and now this disease was asking more of her than she thought she could give.

Unfortunately, I hear this sad story many times a day from wives, daughters and daughters-in-law who are taking care of relatives with Alzheimer's.

While many patients with chronic illnesses require help for a time, Alzheimer's demands much, much more. Caregiving is all-consuming—starting with gentle reminders to someone with a fading memory but transitioning to round-the-clock attention to every aspect of daily life. The vigilance, responsibility and work come at great personal cost to women who are also juggling careers and children. In fact, research shows that the burden of caregiver stress takes a serious emotional and physical toll, increasing the caregiver's own risk for illness and death.

One of the biggest stressors is the stigma attached to the disease. A caregiver told me she stopped going to church on Sundays, because her father spoke out loud at inappropriate moments during the service. She said she feels ostracized by her community, because her father's dementia is so misunderstood. Another caregiver put it this way: "Alzheimer's disease is the new leprosy." We cannot let that attitude take hold, because it divides and isolates us. Women are at the forefront of many societal changes, and now it is time for us to change the public perception of Alzheimer's disease—change from hopeless to hopeful, from alone to supported and incurable to treatable. We can do this in our lifetime.

Physicians can help by diagnosing the disease in its early stages and educating caregivers about what to expect throughout the process. In fact, recent research from the Minneapolis VA Hospital shows that this approach helped "lower family caregivers' anxiety, depression and stress." Indeed, good care management and collaboration between caregivers and medical professionals can lower outpatient healthcare costs by 30 percent.

Caregiving is a job that no one asks for, and support is essential. Alzheimer's is a particularly cruel disease that ultimately robs patients of their ability to make decisions, but it should not rob them of their dignity. Caregivers who have support and who understand the disease process can feel empowered to be the guardians of that dignity.

As a physician, I encourage women to ask others to help—their neighbors, family, faith community or the Alzheimer's Association volunteers.

"It isn't supposed to be like this." No, it is not. Let's work together to change it.

A Woman's Disease

What Toll Does Alzheimer Caregiving Take on Women?

Responding to the Caregiving Crisis

By former First Lady Rosalynn Carter, president of the board of the Rosalynn Carter Institute for Caregiving, which builds support for caregivers worldwide

After having worked in the mental health field for a long time and seeing the hardships family caregivers face day after day caring for a loved one with mental illness, I realized how little help was available for them. That's why when we came home from the White House, we established the Rosalynn Carter Institute for Caregiving at our local state university, Georgia Southwestern.

I quickly learned that we are in the midst of a caregiving crisis in America. Everyone is affected. Thanks to the wonders of medicine and our growing knowledge about the causes of many health problems, so many more of us are living longer and therefore en-countering problems associated with aging. Today, many seniors with some of the most challenging care needs would not have even survived a decade ago due to the severity of their illnesses. Increased longevity means we are also seeing people in their 70s caring for parents in their 90s.

Family caregivers have always been the backbone of our country's long-term care system, and they continue to care for the vast majority of dependent people at home. In the United States, they provide more than twice the amount of unpaid services each year than all the money spent nationwide on nursing homes and paid home care combined. Yet family caregivers are largely neglected by the health and long-term care systems. They frequently are not trained on how to deliver complicated care, not treated as part-ners in their loved one's care, nor encouraged to maintain their own health.

In addition, while our aging population continues to increase rapidly, our professional caregiving workforce is decreasing, leaving family caregivers overwhelmed and ill-equipped to cope with the complex care needs and difficult behaviors associated with chronic illnesses, including Alzheimer's and other dementias. Research shows that fam-ily caregivers are at an increased risk for health, emotional, financial and work-related problems due to the strain of providing care.

The good news is that there are caregiver support programs that work! These evidence-based programs* help caregivers provide high-quality care without becoming ill themselves. They also enable them to provide care at home for longer periods without resorting to institutional care for their loved ones. Sadly, these programs are not currently available in most communities.

> **" I quickly learned that we are in the midst of a caregiving crisis in America. Everyone is affected. "**

We must take the next step and put these programs into practice in real-world community settings. For this to happen in any meaningful way, there must be a call to action to the public, the medical community and policymakers to support our ailing family members and the people who care for them. We need a national policy on caregiver assistance that recognizes the long-term contributions of family caregivers and understands the importance of investing to sustain them.

It's common sense! Comprehensively supporting caregivers results in great cost savings for individual families, Medicaid and private insurance. It also allows individuals to remain in their own homes for longer periods of time. Let's do what it takes to help maintain the health and quality of life for both the caregiver and the ill loved one.

*See the "Evidence-Based Resources" section of the Rosalynn Carter Institute for Caregiving website at www.rosalynncarter.org for details on existing evidence-based programs for caregivers developed by leading researchers in our country.

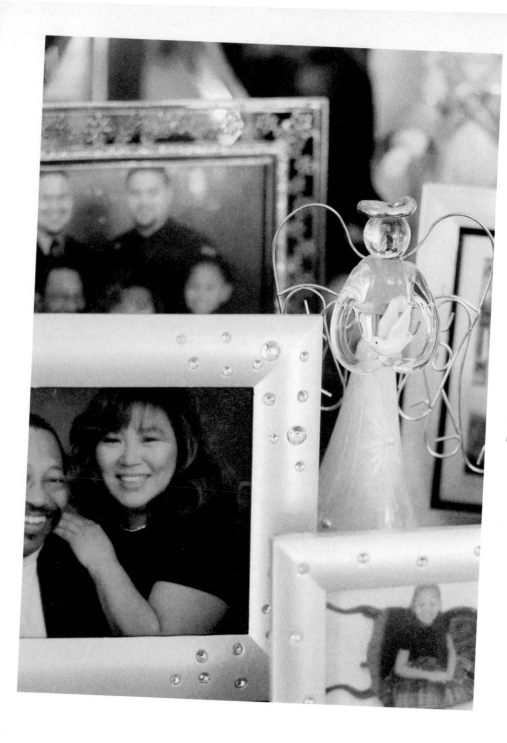

Caring for Alzheimer's
11 Million Different Views

66 It was hard because she thought I was somebody else. The relationship changed over the course of the illness. I actually got along with her better. 99

66 I have grandchildren and I'd like to see them grow up. Sit on a porch where it is warm and be able to tell them stuff that went on. That's something my mother couldn't do. 99

66 When my mother got Alzheimer's she became a nice old lady. Before that, she used to be kind of argumentative. 99

66 They shouldn't keep the families in the dark. They gave her a new medication. They didn't tell us what it was for, but she became hypersexual. It's embarrassing to talk about, but I guess it's a sign of Alzheimer's. 99

From interviews of family members caring for loved ones with Alzheimer's, The Elder Care Study, Families and Work Institute, 2010.

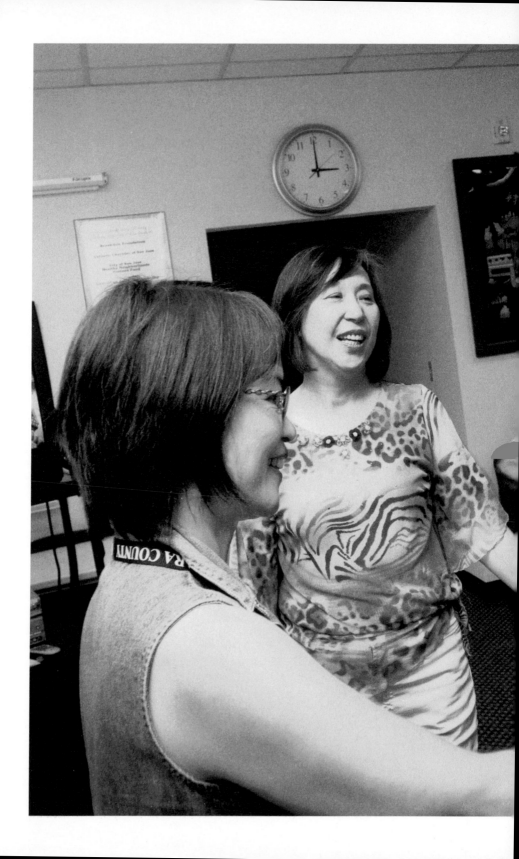

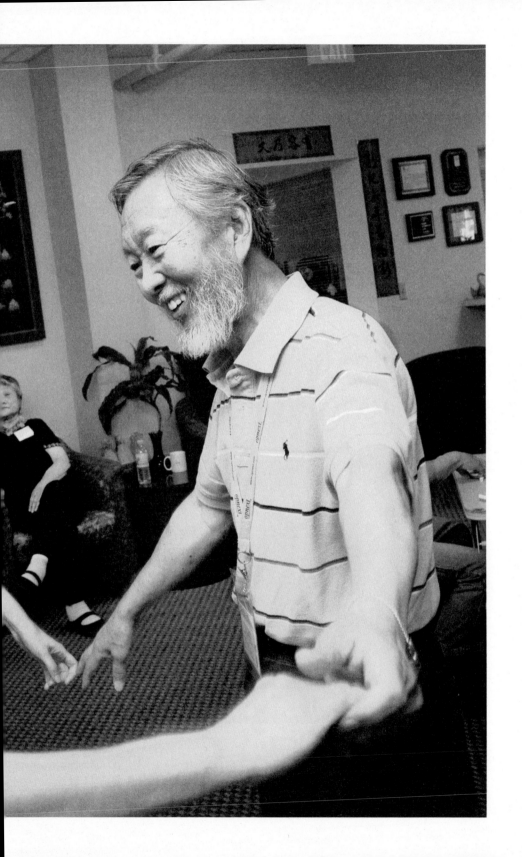

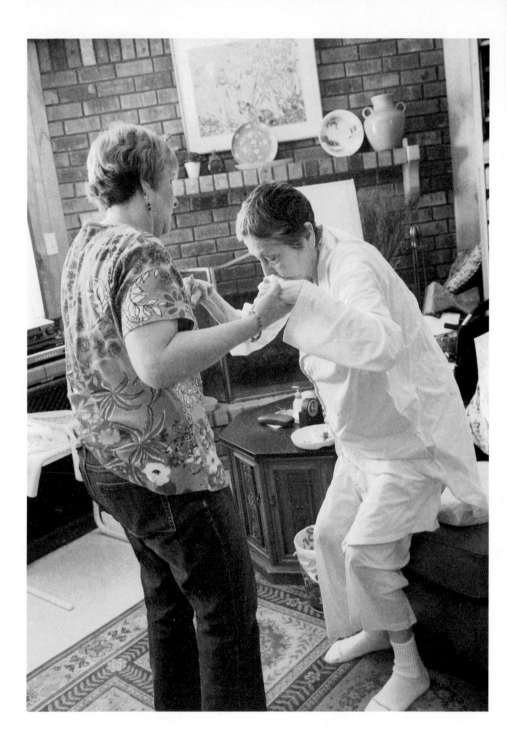

What Toll Does Alzheimer Caregiving Take on Women?

By Dale Fetherling and Sam Fazio, Ph.D., with Katie Maslow

A pioneering new Alzheimer's Association poll paints a surprising and sobering picture of the millions of dedicated women caring for people with Alzheimer's disease. The poll, believed to be the largest ever on Alzheimer's disease, involved interviews with 3,118 adults nationwide, including more than 500 Alzheimer caregivers.

This in-depth poll of male and female caregivers reveals that 60 percent of Alzheimer caregivers are women. Of those women, 68 percent report emotional stress from caregiving—nearly half rate their stress as a "5 on a scale of 1 to 5"—and more than half (51 percent) acknowledge physical stress. (Unless otherwise noted, all poll results in this chapter are from the Alzheimer's Association's 2010 Women and Alzheimer's Poll, the methodology of which is detailed in the Appendix.)

> *Nearly half of women rate their stress around caring for someone with Alzheimer's at the highest level possible.*

Additionally, six out of ten caregivers believe this progressive disease is genetic. Perhaps as a result, 57 percent of all caregivers (including two-thirds of the women) fear getting Alzheimer's themselves. Most caregivers, whether male or female, are very concerned with maintaining their own health.

The decision to become a caregiver—and about four in ten report having no real choice— can have a major impact on the caregivers' lives. Some have had to quit their jobs, and among those who still work, almost two-thirds report having to go in late, leave early or take time off from work to provide care.

But the biggest impact may be on caregivers' relationships. Caregivers report caring for a wide range of relatives and friends, the most common being their mothers. As a result, 46 percent of female caregivers report they are spending less time with their spouse/partner, and another 39 percent say that puts a strain on their marriage. Interestingly, about 10 percent more male Alzheimer caregivers than female ones believe caregiving strains their marriage.

Those and many other facts revealed by the poll help paint a portrait of who these caregivers are, what they do and how caregiving affects them. Supported by a special analysis of 2009 data from a National Alliance for Caregiving/AARP survey of caregiving in the United States as well as other studies, this chapter seeks to present a comprehensive view of caregiving. It looks at not only what price caregivers pay—and what payoff they derive—from their service but also suggests what may be done to help and support them.

Numbers alone, of course, tell only part of the story. In the essays that follow this chapter you will read personal, poignant stories by the caregivers themselves, stories that put flesh and blood on this chapter's statistical bones.

As one essayist writes:

> As the disease progressed, her confusion, disorientation and fear worsened. She was unable to remember what day it was or even the name of our president. Her panic increased, and my own fear and sense of helplessness and guilt became overwhelming. It was a terrible day when we stood together in front of a mirror, and she turned to me and said, "Who are you?"

Another woman, one of the most powerful people in the country, describes a helplessness that many caregivers can appreciate:

> We felt powerless, and we were powerless. Though I was a United States Senator, though I could get the highest levels of the National Institutes of Health on the phone, though I could have a Nobel Prize winner from Johns Hopkins return my call, I could not help my father. No one knew how to slow or stop the course of this terrible disease.

Alzheimer caregiver

The United States is becoming a nation of caregivers, and in a majority of cases (60 percent), female caregivers. The average unpaid Alzheimer caregiver is a white, married working woman over age 50.

About 6.7 million American women now provide unpaid care for a person with Alzheimer's disease or other dementia. That number is not only huge, it is sure to increase as the nation's population ages and the incidence of Alzheimer's grows.

According to this new Alzheimer's Association poll, most caregivers (66 percent) are married, and 44 percent are employed full- or part-time, with the majority (55 percent) being the primary breadwinners of the household. Though men and women report caring for a wide range of relatives and friends, most commonly caregivers attend to their mothers (31 percent) or spouses (15 percent).

As the NAC/AARP study also points out, 70 percent of Alzheimer and dementia caregivers are taking care of a woman (see Fig. 1). The typical recipient of care is female, age 81 and widowed. Thus, in large measure, caregivers for people with Alzheimer's and other dementias consist of women taking care of other women.

FIGURE 1 : Proportion of Care Recipients by Gender, U.S., 2009

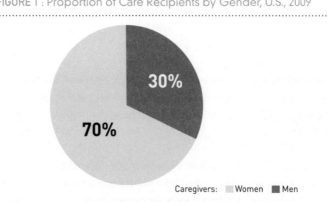

Caregivers: Women   Men

Source: Alzheimer's Association. Unpublished data from the NAC/AARP 2009 survey of caregiving in the United States, prepared under contract by Matthew Greenwald and Associates, 2010.

Why do they become caregivers?

Deciding factors are numerous, but the most common answer (84 percent of women) is to keep their relative or friend at home and out of an institution. (A quarter of women caregivers have promised to keep their loved one out of an institution, though nearly a third fear that promise may need to be broken.)

Other factors women cite as affecting their decision:

- Lack of other family: 58 percent

- Cost of in-home help: 57 percent

- Having no one else you can trust: 56 percent

- Obligation as spouse/partner: 49 percent

- Being the only woman in the family: 39 percent

In fact, more than 41 percent of females agreed with the statement "I had no choice in becoming a caregiver."

Forty-one percent of women caring for someone with Alzheimer's say they didn't have a choice.

Caregiving responsibilities are both long-term and time-intensive. Of female caregivers sampled, nearly two out of five have been providing care for more than five years. And more than three in ten female caregivers live with the person with Alzheimer's and take care of him or her 24/7.

The NAC/AARP study found that female Alzheimer and dementia caregivers provide an average of 24 hours of care a week, compared with 18 hours a week for male Alzheimer and dementia caregivers and 17 hours a week for caregivers of other older people. Actual hours of caregiving vary widely around the 24-hour average: 18 percent of these caregivers provide 41 or more hours of care a week; 10 percent provide 21 to 40 hours; 26 percent provide 9 to 20 hours, and 44 percent provide 8 or fewer hours of care a week.

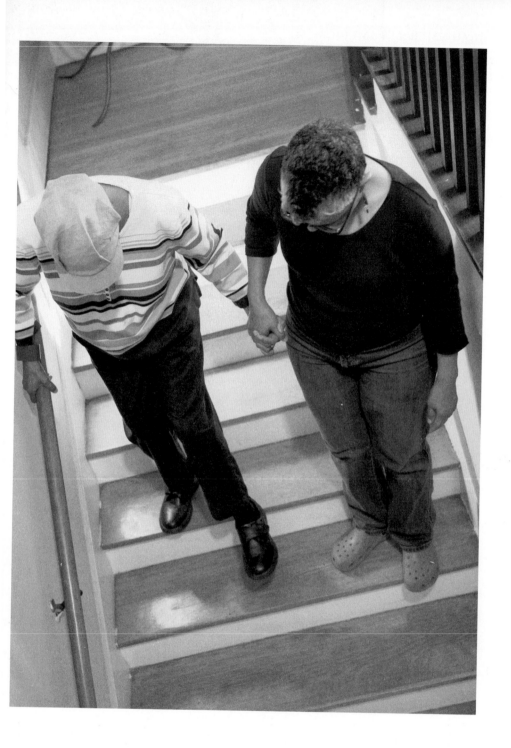

Taking care of loved one with Alzheimer's : Women caregivers have been taking care of someone with Alzheimer's disease longer than men caregivers. Also, a majority of women caring for their loved ones are living with them, compared to a plurality of male caregivers.

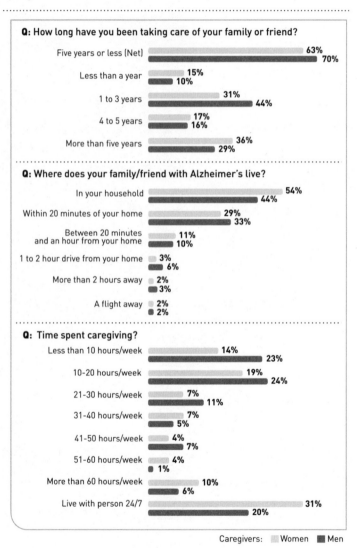

Q: How long have you been taking care of your family or friend?

- Five years or less (Net): 63% / 70%
- Less than a year: 15% / 10%
- 1 to 3 years: 31% / 44%
- 4 to 5 years: 17% / 16%
- More than five years: 36% / 29%

Q: Where does your family/friend with Alzheimer's live?

- In your household: 54% / 44%
- Within 20 minutes of your home: 29% / 33%
- Between 20 minutes and an hour from your home: 11% / 10%
- 1 to 2 hour drive from your home: 3% / 6%
- More than 2 hours away: 2% / 3%
- A flight away: 2% / 2%

Q: Time spent caregiving?

- Less than 10 hours/week: 14% / 23%
- 10-20 hours/week: 19% / 24%
- 21-30 hours/week: 7% / 11%
- 31-40 hours/week: 7% / 5%
- 41-50 hours/week: 4% / 7%
- 51-60 hours/week: 4% / 1%
- More than 60 hours/week: 10% / 6%
- Live with person 24/7: 31% / 20%

Caregivers: Women   Men

Source: Alzheimer's Association, Unpublished data from the NAC/AARP 2009 survey of caregiving in the United States, prepared under contract by Matthew Greenwald and Associates, 2010.

The NAC/AARP study also found that about one-quarter of female caregivers (23 percent) provide care for the person with Alzheimer's or another dementia in the caregiver's home. Slightly more than half (54 percent) provide care for the person in his or her own home or the home of a relative or friend, and the remaining 23 percent provide care for a person who is living in a nursing home, assisted living facility or retirement community. Among female Alzheimer and dementia caregivers who provide care for a person who does not live with them, about half (51 percent) live within 20 minutes of the person; 15 percent live between 20 minutes and an hour from the person; 3 percent live one to two hours from the person, and 8 percent live more than two hours from the person.

What do they do?

Substantial proportions of caregivers of people with Alzheimer's and other dementias provide help with many daily personal care activities, as reported in the NAC/AARP poll (see Fig. 2). Female caregivers are about 25 percent more likely than male caregivers to report that they provide help with the activities shown in the figure, but male caregivers are more likely than female caregivers to say they provide help with two of the activities: getting in and out of bed and chairs, and feeding.

FIGURE 2 : Proportion of Alzheimer and Other Dementia Caregivers Who Provide Help with Personal Care Activities by Gender, U.S., 2009

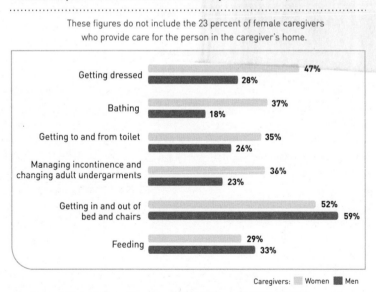

These figures do not include the 23 percent of female caregivers who provide care for the person in the caregiver's home.

Activity	Women	Men
Getting dressed	47%	28%
Bathing	37%	18%
Getting to and from toilet	35%	26%
Managing incontinence and changing adult undergarments	36%	23%
Getting in and out of bed and chairs	52%	59%
Feeding	29%	33%

Caregivers: Women ▨ Men ■

Source: Alzheimer's Association, Unpublished data from the NAC/AARP 2009 survey of caregiving in the United States, prepared under contract by Matthew Greenwald and Associates, 2010.

Decision to become a caregiver: Both sexes agree that keeping a family member/friend at home is the primary reason for becoming a caregiver. On the other hand, women caregivers are much more concerned than men caregivers when considering cost of in-home help.

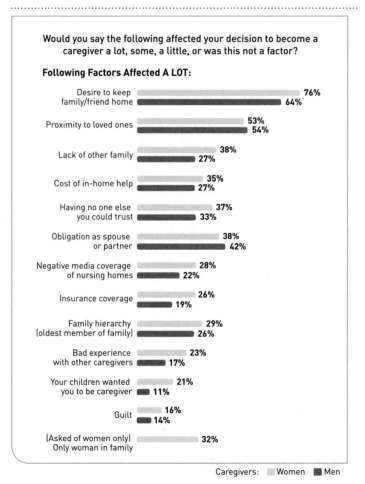

Would you say the following affected your decision to become a caregiver a lot, some, a little, or was this not a factor?

Following Factors Affected A LOT:

Desire to keep family/friend home — 76% / 64%

Proximity to loved ones — 53% / 54%

Lack of other family — 38% / 27%

Cost of in-home help — 35% / 27%

Having no one else you could trust — 37% / 33%

Obligation as spouse or partner — 38% / 42%

Negative media coverage of nursing homes — 28% / 22%

Insurance coverage — 26% / 19%

Family hierarchy (oldest member of family) — 29% / 26%

Bad experience with other caregivers — 23% / 17%

Your children wanted you to be caregiver — 21% / 11%

Guilt — 16% / 14%

(Asked of women only) Only woman in family — 32%

Caregivers: Women ■ Men

Source: Alzheimer's Association. Unpublished data from the NAC/AARP 2009 survey of caregiving in the United States, prepared under contract by Matthew Greenwald and Associates. 2010.

In fact, working women complain that they get even less employer support for elder care than they do for child care. Thirty-eight percent of women workers say it is easier to ask for time off to care for children (50 percent report no difference). Forty-five percent of working-women caregivers (and 36 percent of men) wanted time off for Alzheimer caregiving and could not get it. Half of the working-women caregivers find it easier to find caregiving for children than for people with Alzheimer's.

> *Thirty-eight percent of women workers say it is easier to ask for time off to care for children than elders. Forty-five percent of working-women caregivers (and 36 percent of men) wanted time off for Alzheimer caregiving and could not get it.*

Money

A majority of caregivers (56 percent) feel their family's finances have suffered, including 32 percent who acknowledge "a great deal" of financial suffering. Both men and women caregivers have similar views about the degree to which their finances have been affected.

According to the NAC/AARP survey, more than one-fifth of female Alzheimer and dementia caregivers went from full-time to part-time work, took a less demanding job or gave up work entirely because of caregiving. Those caregivers clearly pay a long-term financial penalty for the time they spend giving care, not only current income and benefits but also contributions to Social Security and other employment-related pension and retirement funds, thus jeopardizing their future financial security.

Relationships

Most (78 percent) caregivers surveyed in the Alzheimer's Association poll, whether men or women, report having less time for friends or family. Almost half of female caregivers (46 percent) report spending less time with their spouse/partner because they are taking care of a friend or relative, and 39 percent say this absence has strained their marriage.

Yet the need to juggle multiple, sometimes conflicting schedules and duties is clear. Almost half of men and women say they need to coordinate schedules with their spouse at least once a day.

Health

Caregiving can ultimately have an impact on the caregivers' health. Nearly seven in ten (68 percent) of women caregivers report emotional stress, and 51 percent cite physical stress from caregiving. Nearly half of the women rate the emotional stress of Alzheimer caregiving at a "5," the highest possible number in the poll.

More specifically, a third of caregiving females feel isolated, and among that group, 16 percent feel depressed and 11 percent feel always tired. And almost half, whether men or women, are very concerned with maintaining their own health.

Caregiving for people with Alzheimer's can also bring with it its own anxiety. About one-quarter of Alzheimer and dementia caregivers have clinically significant anxiety related to caregiving,[1] and female caregivers are more likely than male caregivers to have these symptoms.[2-3] It also appears that the more you know about the disease, the more you fear getting it. More than three-fourths of women caregivers think that if someone from her family gets the disease, "there is a good chance" the caregiver will get Alzheimer's, too.

Many caregivers of people with Alzheimer's and other dementias experience negative physical health effects associated with caregiving. Research shows that Alzheimer and dementia caregivers are more likely than noncaregivers to have high levels of stress hormones,[4, 6] reduced immune function,[4, 7-10] slow wound healing,[11] new hypertension,[12] increased levels of D-dimer, a risk factor for cardiovascular disease,[13] and new coronary heart disease.[14]

These negative health effects are generally attributed to emotional stress caused by caregiving. In addition, some caregivers neglect their own health, saying, for example, that they don't have enough time or energy for exercise or doctor appointments for their own health conditions.[15] Some caregivers also experience physical strain associated with caregiving. In response to the NAC/AARP survey, 24 percent of female Alzheimer and dementia caregivers reported that they experience physical strain as a result of caregiving.[16] Smaller proportions of male Alzheimer and dementia caregivers (12 percent) and

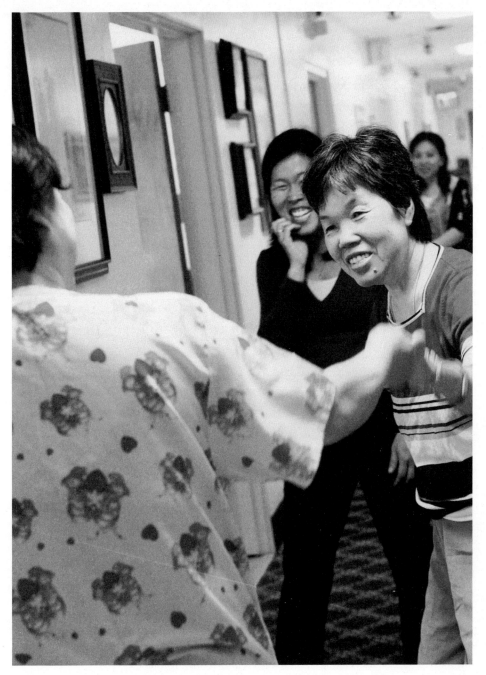

My Quach, far right, has been living with Alzheimer's disease for seven years.

caregivers of other older people (19 percent) said they experience physical strain because of caregiving.

More than half of Alzheimer and dementia caregivers say they feel that they have to be "on duty" 24 hours a day in order to anticipate and prevent problems and ensure the person's safety.[17-18] This need for 24-hour vigilance contributes to caregiver stress and anxiety and affects caregivers of people in all stages of dementia, including those who are in the late stages of dementia and permanently placed in a nursing home[19] and those who are in the very early stages of dementia and may be at risk of wandering and getting lost or other unsafe activities.[20]

> *Three-quarters of all caregivers are concerned about their own health since becoming a caregiver.*

Also, some studies have found that caregivers of older people, including people with Alzheimer's and other dementias, are more likely than non-caregivers to develop cognitive impairment.[21-24] These studies also show that the cognitive impairment is associated with emotional stress,[23] depression and elevated stress hormones.[24]

Caregiver gender gaps

Though men and women caregivers often responded in parallel fashion to the poll's questions, the disparity in their answers is striking in several cases. One of the largest differences came in relation to being "frightened" of getting Alzheimer's disease. Women are much more fearful, most notably about the prospect of becoming a burden to their families. Men, on the other hand, most fear not being able to take care of themselves (such as bathing, cooking and other simple chores) and forgetting who their loved ones are.

Women caregivers are substantially more likely to live with the person with Alzheimer's and take care of them 24/7 than are male caregivers. Females are much more physically stressed by caregiving than men, and they place a significantly higher importance to caring for parents and for keeping the extended family living together.

If they themselves developed Alzheimer's, more women than men would prefer to have paid caregivers take care of them at home. But slightly more men would opt to be taken care of by their spouse or children or be placed in an assisted-living home that specializing in caring for people with Alzheimer's.

The upside

Most Alzheimer and dementia caregivers appear to experience some positive effects of caregiving. For instance, about seven in ten state they have a friend, family, religious or community group that offers them support. They count on support networks, including family (25 percent), friends (12 percent) and faith (17 percent) while a smaller percentage (7 percent) use recreation or other activities to help them cope.

According to one caregiver:

> *Who's to say that my mother's Alzheimer's won't help my own memory— remind me of who I was raised to be, who I really am?*

The positive effects and the words caregivers use to describe them vary from one caregiver to another but often include: finding a sense of meaning or purpose in their lives; feeling useful; feeling good about fulfilling vows and obligations or being able to "give back" to someone who took care of them; taking pride in being able to manage difficult situations; feeling strong and capable; and enjoying being with (or specific aspects of being with) the person.[25-27]

What can be done to help?

Despite such positive effects, it is clear that most caregivers experience the task as difficult and debilitating. Caregivers in the poll showed themselves to be especially well informed and very concerned about the disease.

The policy implications from their answers suggest they:

- overwhelmingly want more research.

- would prefer placement in a care facility specializing in Alzheimer's if they themselves developed the disease.

- want—even more than time off from work—paid-care options, such as adult day centers or respite care providers.

There is little evidence that those objectives are being vigorously met. However, the discussion in this chapter does underscore how those and other efforts might be made to help Alzheimer and dementia caregivers:

- Caregiver assessment should precede efforts to assist. The many differences among caregivers and caregiving situations mean that it is essential to understand each caregiver's situation before trying to identify ways to support that caregiver. Public and private agencies that provide services for people with Alzheimer's and other dementias should be aware of this heterogeneity and ask caregivers explicitly about their caregiving situation. Many public programs that pay for services for people with Alzheimer's and other dementias currently do not routinely assess the caregiver, thus implying wrongly that a "one size fits all" approach in terms of services will be effective in widely diverse caregiving situations.[28]

- Programs found to be feasible should be made widely available. Programs that can increase caregivers' satisfaction with social support and self-efficacy are likely to reduce the negative effects of caregiving. Many such programs have been shown to achieve these goals in carefully conducted research. Eight of these programs and their demonstrated outcomes are listed in Box 1. At present, federal government agencies, including the U.S. Administration on Aging and the U.S. Department of Veterans Affairs, and private organizations, such as the Rosalynn Carter Institute, are funding projects to test the feasibility of providing these programs in local communities.

- Paid services should be available in every community. These services, such as adult day care, home care and respite services, can help individual caregivers. Financial support should be provided for caregivers who cannot afford the services themselves.

- Workplace policies that can help caregivers should be implemented widely. Family caregiver leave policies, including paid leave and greater flexibility in work hours could greatly benefit all caregivers, including particularly, the adult daughters, daughters-in-law and granddaughters who are juggling multiple parenting, work and caregiving responsibilities.

To better prepare for the effect of this rapidly growing disease, it will be crucial to understand what is asked of caregivers, how they respond and what more we can to do help them cope and provide the best possible care for their loved ones.

BOX 1: 8 Programs That Have Been Shown to Help Caregivers
of People with Alzheimer's Disease and Other Dementias

The Anger and Depression Management Program is shown to
reduce caregiver depression and increase caregiver
self-efficacy.[29]

**The Cleveland Alzheimer's Managed Care Demonstration
Program** is shown to reduce caregiver depression.[30]

The Home Environmental Skill Building Program is shown to
reduce caregiver stress, reduce caregiver upset about the care
recipient's behavioral symptoms, decrease care recipient
behavioral symptoms, and increase caregiver self-efficacy for
female caregivers.[31-32]

The New York University Caregiver Intervention Program is shown
to reduce caregiver depression, reduce caregiver upset about
the care recipient's behavioral symptoms, improve social
support and improve caregiver self-rated health.[33-36]

The Progressively Lowered Stress Threshold Program is shown to
reduce caregiver stress and depression, reduce caregiver
upset about the care recipient's behavioral symptoms and
improve caregiver immune function.[37-40]

**The Resources for Enhancing Alzheimer's Caregiver Health
(REACH II) Program** is shown to reduce caregiver depression,
decrease care recipient behavioral symptoms, improve social
support and improve caregiver self-rated health.[41-42]

The Savvy Caregiver Program is shown to reduce caregiver stress
and depression, and reduce caregiver upset about the care
recipient's behavioral symptoms.[43-44]

The STAR-C Program is shown to reduce caregiver stress and
depression, reduce caregiver upset about the care recipient's
behavioral symptoms, and decrease care recipient behavioral
symptoms.[45]

ENDNOTES

1   C. Cooper; T.B.S. Balamorali and G. Livingston, "A Systematic Review of the Prevalence and Covariates of Anxiety in Caregivers of People with Dementia," *International Psychogeriatrics* 2007;19(2):175-195.

2   R. Schulz and L.M. Martire, "Family Caregiving of Persons with Dementia: Prevalence, Health Effects, and Support Strategies," *American Journal of Geriatric Psychiatry* 2004;12:3:240-249.

3   M.A. Lieberman and L. Fisher, "The Impact of Chronic Illness on the Health and Well-Being of Family Members," *Gerontologist* 1995:35(1):94-102.

4   S.K. Lutgendorf; L. Garand; K.C. Buckwalter; T.T. Reimer; S-Y Hong and D.M. Lubaroff, "Life Stress, Mood Disturbance, and Elevated Interleukin-6 in Healthy Older Women," *Journal of Gerontology: Medical Sciences* 1999;54A(9):M434-439.

5   J.K. Kiecolt-Glaser; R. Glaser; S. Gravenstein; W.B. Malarkey and J. Sheridan, "Chronic Stress Alters the Immune Response to Influenza Virus Vaccine in Older Adults," *Proceedings of the National Academy of Sciences* 1996;93:3043-3047.

6   R. von Kanel, J.E. Dimsdale; P.J. Mills; S. Ancoli-Israel; T.L.Patterson; B.T. Mausback, et al., "Effect of Alzheimer Caregiving Stress and Age on Frailty Markers Interleukin-6, C-Reactive Protein, and D-Diner," *Journal of Gerontology: Medical Sciences* 2006;61A(9):963-969.

7   M.E. Bauera, K. Vedharaab, P. Perksa, G.K. Wilcockc, S.L. Lightmana and N. Shanksa, "Chronic Stress in Caregivers of Dementia Patients is Associated with Reduced Lymphocyte Sensitivity to Glucocorticoids," *Journal of Neuroimmunology* 2000;103(1):84-92.

8   J.K. Kiecolt-Glaser; J.R. Dura; C.E. Speicher; O.J. Trask and R. Galser, "Spousal Caregivers of Dementia Victims: Longitudinal Changes in Immunity and Health," *Psychosomatic Medicine* 1991;53:345-362.

9   P.J. Mills; H. Yu; M.G. Ziegler; T. Patterson and I. Grant, "Vulnerable Caregivers of Patients with Alzheimer's Disease Have a Deficit in Circulating CD62L T Lymphocytes," *Psychosomatic Medicine* 1999;61:168-174.

10 P.G. Mills, K.A. Adler, J.E. Dimsdale, C. Perez, M.G. Ziegler, S. Ancoli-Israel, et al., "Vulnerable Caregivers of Alzheimer Disease Patients Have a Deficit in [beta]2–Adrenergic Receptor Sensitivity and Density," *American Journal of Geriatric Psychiatry* 2004;12(3):281-286.

11 J.K. Kiecolt-Glaser, P.T. Marucha PT; Mercado AM; Malarkey WB; and Glaser R. "Slowing of Wound Healing by Psychological Stress," *Lancet* 1995;346(8984):1194-1196.

12 W.S. Shaw; T.L. Patterson; M.G. Ziegler; J.E. Dimsdale; S.J. Semple and I. Grant, "Accelerated Risk of Hypertensive Blood Pressure Recordings among Alzheimer Caregivers," *Journal of Psychosomatic Research* 1999;46(3):215-227.

13 R. von Kanel, J.E. Dimsdale, K.A. Adler, T.L. Patterson, P.J. Mills and I. Grant, "Exaggerated Plasma Fibrin Formation (D-dimer) in Elderly Alzheimer Caregivers as Compared to Noncaregiving Controls," *Gerontology* 2005;51(1):7-13.

14 P.P. Vitaliano; J.M. Scanlan J. Zhang, M.V. Savage, I.B. Hirsch and I. Siegler, "A Path Model of Chronic Stress, the Metabolic Syndrome, and Coronary Heart Disease," *Psychosomatic Medicine* 2002;64:418-435.

15 L.C. Burton, B. Zdaniuk, R. Schulz, S. Jackson and C. Hirsch, "Transitions in Spousal Caregiving," *Gerontologist* 2003;43(2):230-241.

16 Alzheimer's Association. Unpublished data from the 2009 National Alliance for Caregiving (NAC)/AARP survey of caregiving in the United States, prepared under contract for the Alzheimer's Association by Matthew Greenwald and Associates, April 8, 2010.

17 D.F. Mahoney, R.N. Jones; D.W. Coon; A.B. Mendelsohn, L.N. Gitlin and M. Ory, "The Caregiver Vigilance Scale, Application and Validation in the Resources for Enhancing Alzheimer's Caregiver Health (REACH) Project," *American Journal of Alzheimer's Disease and Other Dementias* 2003;18(1):39-48.

18 R. Schulz, A.B. Mendelsohn; W.E. Haley; D. Mahoney; R.S. Allen; S. Zhang, et al., "End-of-Life Care and the Effects of Bereavement on Family Caregivers of Persons with Dementia," *New England Journal of Medicine* 2003;349(20):1936-42. .

19 D.F. Mahoney, "Vigilance, Evolution and Definition for Caregivers of Family Members with Alzheimer's Disease," *Journal of Gerontological Nursing* 2003;29(8):24-30.

20 K.B. Adams, "The Transition to Caregiving: The Experience of Family Members Embarking on the Dementia Caregiving Career," *Journal of Gerontological Social Work* 2006;47(3/4):3-29.

21 I.W. Caswell, P.P Vitaliano, K.L. Croyle, J.M. Scanlan; J. Zhang and A. Daruwala, "Negative Associations of Chronic Stress and Cognitive Performance in Older Adult Spouse Caregivers," *Experimental Aging Research* 2003;29(3):202-318.

22 S. Lee, I. Kawachi and F. Grodstein," Does Caregiving Stress Affect Cognitive Function in Older Women?" *Journal of Nervous and Mental Disease* 2004;192(1):51-57.

23 C.S. Mackenzie, U.J. Wiprzycha, L. Hasher and D. Goldstein, "Associations Between Psychological Distress, Learning, and Memory in Spouse Caregivers of Older Adults," *Journal of Gerontology, Psychological Sciences* 2009;64B(6):742-746.

24 P.P. Vitaliano; J. Zhang, H.M. Young; I..W. Caswell, J.M. Scanlan and D. Echeverria, "Depressed Mood Mediates Decline in Cognitive Processing Speed in Caregivers," *Gerontologist* 2009;49(1):12-22.

25 C.J. Farran; B.H. Miller; J.E. Kaufman and L. Davis, "Race, Finding Meaning, and Caregiver Distress," *Journal of Aging and Health* 1997;9(3):316-333.

26 B.J. Kramer, "Gain in the Caregiving Experience: Where are We? What Next?" *Gerontologist* 1997;37(2):218-232.

27 B.J. Tarlow, S.R. Wisniewski, S.H. Belle, M. Rubert, M.G. Ory and D. Gallagher-Thompson, "Positive Aspects of Caregiving: Contributions of the REACH Project to the Development of New Measures for Alzheimer's Caregiving," *Research on Aging* 2004;26(4):429-453.

28 Family Caregiver Alliance. *Caregiver Assessment: Principles, Guidelines and Strategies for Change: Report from a National Consensus Development Conference.* (San Francisco, CA: 2006).

29 D.W. Coon, L. Thompson, A. Steffen, K. Sorocco and D. Gallagher-Thompson, "Anger and Depression Management: Psychoeducational Skill Training Interventions For Women Caregivers of a Relative with Dementia," *Gerontologist* 2003;43(5):678-689.

30 D.M. Bass, P.A. Clark, W.J. Looman, C.A. McCarthy and S. Eckert, "The Cleveland Alzheimer's Managed Care Demonstration: Outcomes after 12 Months of Implementation," *Gerontologist* 2003;43(1):73-85.

31 L.N. Gitlin, L. Winter, M. Corcoran, M.P. Dennis, S. Schinfeld and W.W. Hauck, "Effects of the Home Environmental Skill-Building Program on the Caregiver–Care Recipient Dyad: 6-Month Outcomes from the Philadelphia REACH Initiative," *Gerontologist* 2003;43(4):532-546.

32 L.N. Gitlin, W.W. Hauck, M.P. Dennis and L. Winter, "Maintenance of Effects of the Home Environmental Skill-Building Program for Family Caregivers and Individuals with Alzheimer's Disease and Related Disorders," *Journals of Gerontology: Biological and Medical Sciences* 2005;60:368-374.

33 P. Drentea, O.J. Clay, D.L. Roth and M.S. Mittelman, "Predictors of Improvement in Social Support: Five-Year Effects of a Structured Intervention for Caregivers of Spouses with Alzheimer's Disease," *Social Science and Medicine* 2006;63:957-967.

34 M.S. Mittelman, S.H. Ferris, E. Shulman, M.A. Steinberg, A. Ambinder, J.A. Mackell, et al., "A Comprehensive Support Program: Effect on Depression in Spouse-Caregivers of AD Patients," *Gerontologist* 1995,35(6):792-802.

35 M.S. Mittelman, D.L. Roth, O.J. Clay and W.E. Haley, "Preserving Health of Alzheimer's Caregivers: Impact of a Spouse Caregiver Intervention," *American Journal of Geriatric Psychiatry* 2007;15(9):780-789.

36 M.S. Mittelman, D.L. Roth, D.W. Coon and W.E. Haley, "Sustained Benefit of Supportive Intervention for Depressive Symptoms in Caregivers of Patients with Alzheimer's Disease," *American Journal of Psychiatry* 2004,161:850-856.

37 K.C. Buckwalter, L. Gerdner, F. Kohout, G.R. Hall, A. Kelly, B. Richards, et al., "A Nursing Intervention to Decrease Depression in Family Caregivers of Persons with Dementia," *Archives of Psychiatric Nursing* 1999;13(2):80-88.

38 L. Garand, K.C. Buckwalter, D.M. Lubaroff, T. Tripp-Reimer, R.A. Frantz and T.N. Ansley, "A Pilot Study of Immune and Mood Outcomes of a Community-Based Intervention for Dementia Caregivers: The PLST Intervention," *Archives of Psychiatric Nursing* 2002;16:156-167.

39 L.A. Gerdner, K.C. Buckwalter and D. Reed, "Impact of a Psychoeducational Nursing Intervention on Frequency of and Response to Behavioral Problems and Functional Decline in Dementia," *Nursing Research* 2002;51(6):363-374.

40 J.M. Stolley, D. Reed and K.C. Buckwalter, "Caregiving Appraisal and Interventions Based on the Progressively Lowered Stress Threshold Model," *American Journal of Alzheimer's Disease and Other Dementias* 2002;17(2):110-120.

41 S.H. Belle, L. Burgio, R. Burns, D. Coon, S.J. Czaja, D. Gallagher-Thompson, et al., "Enhancing the Quality of Life of Dementia Caregivers from Different Ethnic or Racial Groups," *Annals of Internal Medicine* 2006;145(10):727-738.

42 A.F. Elliott, L.D. Burgio and J. DeCoster, "Enhancing Caregiver Health: Findings from the Resources for Enhancing Alzheimer's Caregiver Health II Intervention," *Journal of the American Geriatrics Society* 2010;58(1):30-37.

43 K.W. Hepburn, J. Tornatore, B. Center and S.W.I. Ostwald, "Dementia Family Caregiver Training: Affecting Beliefs about Caregiving and Caregiver Outcomes," *Journal of the American Geriatrics Society* 2001;49(4), 450-457.

44 S.K. Ostwald, K.W. Hepburn, W. Caron, T. Burns and R. Mantell, "Reducing Caregiver Burden: A Randomized Psychoeducational Intervention for Caregivers of Persons with Dementia," *Gerontologist* 1999;39(3), 299-309.

45 L. Teri, S.M. McCurry, R. Logsdon, et al., "Training community consultants to help family members improve dementia care: A randomized controlled trial," *Gerontologist* 2005:45(6):802-811.

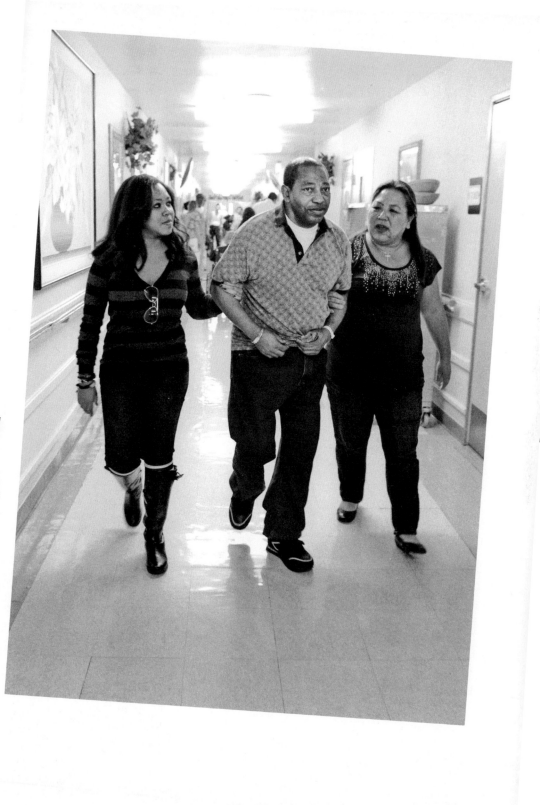

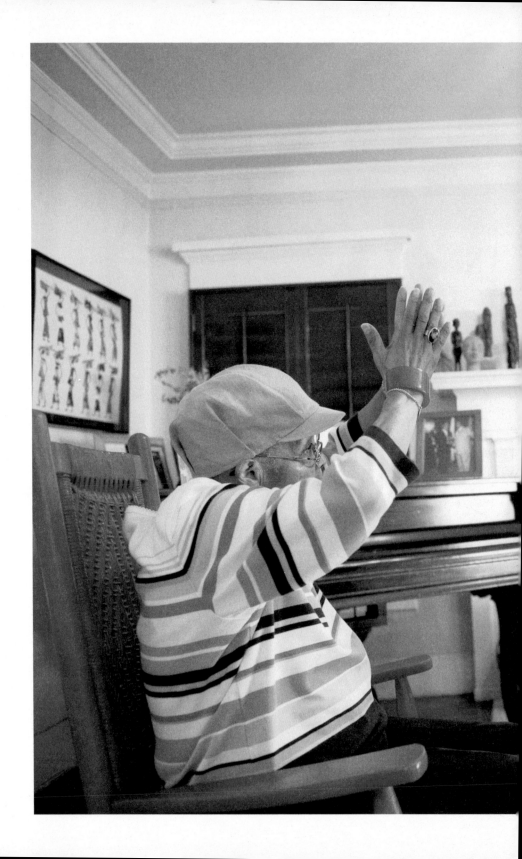

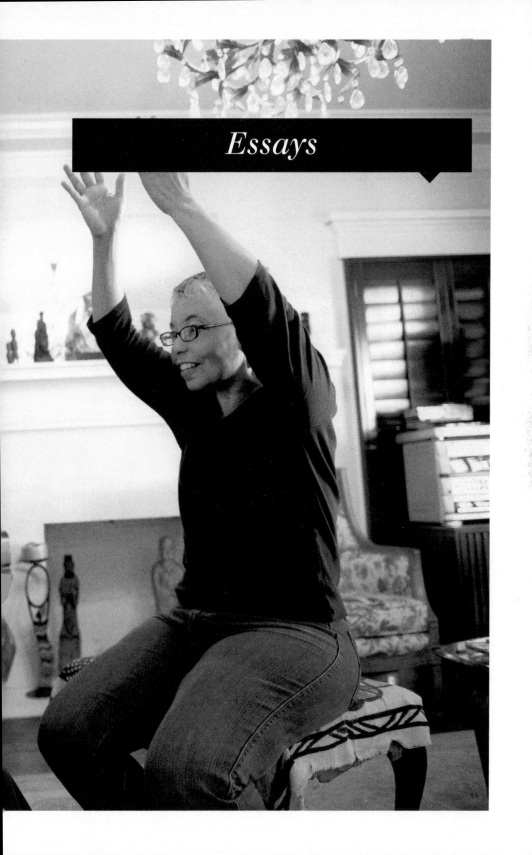

Essays

A Latino Family's Struggle with Alzheimer's

By Beatriz Terrazas, a journalist whose work has appeared in
The Washington Post, The Dallas Morning News *and* More *magazine*

*M*y friend asked the question during a conversation about my mother, who has Alzheimer's: What about a nursing home? She asked because I was on my way to El Paso to relieve my sister for two weeks. My sister works full-time, but she's in charge of scheduling Mom's care. She ferries her to doctor and dentist appointments and back and forth between their homes. It's a tough job, which is why periodically I step in to help.

So why not a nursing home? I gave my friend my standard answer: Residential care isn't an option now for two reasons. One, my mother's dementia doesn't warrant it yet. And two, I worry about the quality of the residential care available to her because she's far below the poverty level guidelines.

Harder to explain, however, is the cultural taboo I keep running into—a wall of intertwined cultures I cannot circumvent. I grapple with it privately.

I'm an American of Mexican descent, born into a family still living largely in Juárez and El Paso. The foundation of my upbringing was twofold: be respectful and be of service, especially to our elders. *Tías, tíos, abuelas, abuelos*—all merit my respect simply because they're older than me. We don't dream of talking back to them, of entering their homes without a proper greeting. Above all, we care for our elderly at home, and they die at home. I remember holding the *rosario* for my grandmother— candles, flowers and the ataúd, her casket—right in her living room in Juárez.

Yes, that was a different time, an era of multigenerational families living, if not under one roof, at least in the same neighborhood. We would even cross the international border at a moment's notice if a family member needed us, al sur or al norte. There was always someone to sit with a housebound loved one. We did it out of duty but also out of love.

I was born in the United States and drank deeply of the American Dream Kool-Aid: You can be anything you want to be, do anything you want to do! There's a lot of good in that dream. It contributes to our country's greatness, our global leadership in science, medicine, technology. But our modern society has also distorted the dream, so that we often seek self-fulfillment at the cost of anything and everyone else. On top of that, we're a youth-venerating culture that's increasingly uncomfortable with anything reminding us of our own old age or mortality. This makes it easy for us to immediately jump to the nursing home solution when faced with sick or elderly family members. Out of sight, out of mind.

> **❝ I sometimes wish there were a different way to care for my mother—one that doesn't cost me work time and wages to be with her. ❞**

The American in me fails miserably sometimes in the service to my mother. I sometimes wish there were a different way to care for her—one that doesn't cost me work time and wages to be with her, one that doesn't involve laying my own wants aside for her needs. Then the Mexican in me says, "Remember where you come from. She's your mother, an elder. *Familia* is about stepping up to the plate. Now just go do it!" It's push and pull.

The friends who bring up the nursing home option are good, family oriented people. They're seeing kids through school, paying college tuition. They're fulfilled by laying aside their own dreams for their children, devoting themselves to shaping good adult human beings. And they are better people for it. If only they could view my journey through the child-rearing prism they know so well. It might help them understand the place I'm coming from.

But maybe they also have a lesson for me. Maybe there's something I'm meant to learn by temporarily laying aside my own wants in order to care for my mother. Perhaps self-fulfillment at this point in my life will come at least partly from the time I spend in service to my her. Who's to say this isn't going to shape my soul into what it was meant to be? Who's to say that my mother's Alzheimer's won't help my own memory and remind me of who I was raised to be, who I really am?

"It's a Family Disease"

By the family of Louise George: daughter Phyllis George, pioneering female sportscaster and former Miss America and First Lady of Kentucky; granddaughter Pamela Brown, WJLA-TV reporter/anchor in Washington, D.C.; and son Rob George, construction company executive in Dallas

Daughter Phyllis

My mother, Louise, died of the insidious disease called Alzheimer's. She was my best friend. Seven years later, the pain still runs through me.

When I was told Mother's dementia was Alzheimer's, I was stunned. Maybe I shouldn't have been, but I realize now my wonderful dad had been covering for her memory problems for years. She really went fast after my father's death in recovery after bypass surgery.

Alzheimer's was the dreaded diagnosis, but the course the disease would take was a mystery. Like millions of other families, my brother Rob and I and our children were embarking on a journey into the unknown, and it felt like we were alone. What was happening to our beautiful, intelligent, caring and loving mother and grandmother? And what was going to happen?

I wanted to protect my children, Pamela and Lincoln, but they could see the pain on my face and in my body. They had never seen me depressed, and now I cried every night before I went to bed and every morning when I got up.

For maybe the first time in my life, I felt helpless. I had always been the "fixer," trying to make things nice for everyone, especially my loved ones. But now I didn't know how to make it better. Pamela would say, "Mom, what's wrong with Grammy?" But I couldn't shield her from it or explain what was happening or teach her how to deal with it. How could I teach her, when my knees buckled under me the first time my mother asked me, "And who are you?"

The truth is, you can read all you want about Alzheimer's, but nothing prepares you for the moments when the consequences of this disease are in your face. And I'm not just talking about the loss of memory that can never be recovered. I'm talking about:

- the blank face devoid of emotion
- the constant repetition of stories over and over again
- the lack of desire to do anything
- the lack of personal hygiene
- the wandering away and getting lost
- the insistent jabbering that sounds like no language on earth
- the so-called Sundowners Syndrome trapping my mother every evening under a dark veil of agitation and confusion

It was so hard to watch, to process, to absorb. All her life, my mother had a stunning appearance, a brilliant mind. She graduated from college when she was 19! She had been the family Rock, the Stabilizer. She loved us so much, took care of us so well. She always told us, "Do what you do to the best of your ability."

So I did my best to shake off the denial and depression. I had to, because I had to be the strong one. I was Mother's primary caregiver—a long-distance primary caregiver and decision-maker, because I was working in New York and Mother lived in Texas. I went on a crash course to learn as much as I could about this horrific disease.

I was determined to give my mother the dignity she so deserved. I brought Bogie, her beloved golden retriever, to visit. I made sure she went to the hair salon once a week. I made sure her pocketbook was next to her bed, so she wouldn't keep searching frantically, "Where's my purse? I need my purse!" That was her security blanket. I put family pictures all around, hoping they would trigger her memory. Most of all, I made sure she had loving caregivers who knew about the disease, whether in a care facility or back at home.

And I coped. When she would call me "Phyl," her nickname for me, I hoped she was coming back. Of course she wasn't. One night after she had broken her hip, I came into her room to find her trying to get out of bed. She looked caught, like a deer in the headlights.

"I want to go home. I want to go home! Take me home!"

I said, "Mother, you have a broken hip. You can't walk."

I will never forget the haunted look on her face when she said, "I've been walking up and down the halls all day!"

Eventually I learned to think of her mind like a lightbulb flickering on and off. When it's on, enjoy the light, appreciate the light, because those moments are few and far between.

It was a long road for us, eight years long. My mother died peacefully with the help and support of kind and compassionate hospice nurses. I thank God for my incredible friends who were there to lean on. Now it was time to grab tight on to the decades of wonderful memories we all shared as a family. Time to let my mother go. Time to let the Alzheimer's go.

But I can't. I will continue to work as a passionate advocate for Alzheimer families. And I pray every day that researchers will find ways to prevent and cure Alzheimer's, so others don't have to experience the fear, the hurt and the pain we went through and still do today.

It's a devastating disease. It's a hideous disease. It's a family disease.

Granddaughter Pamela

I knew my grandmother had Alzheimer's, and I knew that was something horrible. But the reality didn't hit until the day Grammy turned to me and said, "Who are you? What's your name?" It was a punch to the gut.

My grandmother was diagnosed with Alzheimer's when I was a freshman at UNC-Chapel Hill. I felt so helpless knowing she was slowly deteriorating and the emotional toll this took on my mother. It seemed like Mom was always on a flight from New York down to Texas to check on Grammy.

Alzheimer's disease alters your vision. Through our lens, we saw a strong, smart and beautiful woman fading away, her memory and her connections to us disappearing. Through her lens, the view varied depending on the day. Some days she saw us as her family taking care of her. Some days we were strangers to her. And then there were the terrible days when she saw us as enemies conspiring against her. We quickly had to realize this wasn't Grammy. This was the disease talking.

I remember thinking how cruel this Alzheimer's is. It's a thief with an insatiable appetite for all that is precious, pure and meaningful.

It devoured my grandmother, who had lived with such elegance, eloquence and dignity. It tore up my mother, who had done everything she could her whole life to make her own mother proud. It terrorized my brother and me, who wanted to be able to "fix" it but could do nothing to slow down or change one thing that was happening.

If there is something positive that Alzheimer's gave me, it was a tremendous amount of respect for my own mother, who showed me what it truly means to be a loving caregiver. But mostly it was a terrible and terrifying experience. Alzheimer's stripped us all to the core.

My grandmother eventually passed, her Alzheimer's leaving all of us changed forever.

Son Rob

I try to not think about it. But here are my words. This is how it felt back then.

Dawn is coming. The sun will rise and peak. I now know my mother never will rise again. But still, every morning when the sun comes, I think maybe this will be the day she will know me. This will be the day I can tell her one last time that I love her, and she'll hear me. But in my heart, I know it's over.

My nature is to put bad things out of my mind. But this one will not leave. How can this be happening to my mother, a woman so strong, so intelligent, so firm in her beliefs? She now lies there in wait. Is she suffering? In her innermost mind, in her spirit, does she know me? Does she hear me? Does she know that I love her and I miss who she was? While she was "alive," did I express my love and appreciation to her for all she did for me?

Now dusk has come once again.

Will the sun rise and peak tomorrow?

"No, son. It won't"

"Goodbye, Mom. I love you."

Emotional Roller Coaster

By Rosalie Ingrande Asaro of San Diego, who married her husband in 1951

I was calm when I heard the diagnosis from the staff sitting around the table at the University of California, San Diego, Alzheimer's Center. It was no surprise. My husband, Ben, was a very healthy 84-year-old in 2005, but his mind had been slipping away for several years. In the back of my own mind, I dreaded what lay ahead.

I hoped to care for Ben at home until he died. That worked for a while, but it was tough. He slept away hours of the day, waking up drenched and befuddled. He resisted my efforts to get him to change pajamas or shower or eat. He was resistant and belligerent. He sneered when our younger daughter came over, accusing her of planning to steal our house. He screamed mercilessly at my older daughter's little dog he used to love. He grew agitated and disoriented, saying he had to get out of there, had to go home. He was at home.

In the early months, I tried running out to do errands while he was home asleep. But the few times he woke up alone were so frightening, I stopped. I hired a caretaker to help out, but that didn't work either. Ben tried to hit the young man, one day locking him out of the house. The caretaker quit. I gave up. I quit the community theatre company where I'd acted for years. I quit my job in sales. And I stopped going to mass. I was officially housebound.

We had always had a volatile relationship, Ben and I, but through more than a half-century of marriage, we always communicated—at high decibel levels sometimes, but it was communication. That's why it was so hard to accept that I just couldn't reason with him. Often frustrated, I wound up yelling at him. Of course, he yelled back.

One particularly explosive day, I couldn't take any of it anymore. I yelled and cried and accused him of slowly killing me with his Alzheimer's. This time my daughters were witnesses, and they insisted it was finally time for me to relinquish my caregiver role. Once again, I gave up. We placed Ben in a board-and-care facility that week.

The girls would go visit Ben occasionally, but the grandchildren visited even less. Their Papa—who had bestowed on them all the affection and attention he withheld from his own children—didn't resemble this 95-pound, confused old man in the bed. And he couldn't figure out who they were, either.

I went regularly, of course, out of guilt and out of love. Sure, Ben and I had slugged it out verbally all those years, but we had so many good times, too. We loved to travel together, we loved Sinatra and the Rat Pack. We loved to dance at our many relatives' weddings, and we loved playing cards at home with our closest friends until the wee hours.

Ben and I had always laughed as hard as we had fought, and I was unexpectedly reminded of that one day, as I was getting ready to leave the facility. I was looking around for my purse, when Ben asked me with his trademark droll sense of humor, "Are you leaving behind anything besides me?"

The next year and a half was endless. One day, my daughters found him propped up in his wheelchair in the big kitchen, the caregivers trying to feed him. The girls took his hands and they cried, as their father smiled weakly and whispered, "My daughters." There was no more anger, no more confusion—just sweetness. They still hold on to that memory.

In those last months, I told Ben stories about our good times together and the people we shared our life with. I told him about the new neighbors and the election of our country's first African-American president. I told him I loved him, that we all loved him.

Recently, I went through Ben's closet to pack up all his nice clothes to give away. I cried like I haven't cried in months. It still strikes me so strange that this man who stood beside me for so long, so handsome in those same suits, is no longer beside me. But I'm also so grateful that most of my memories of Ben are from the days when he was strong and funny and healthy.

I've been back at work for more than a year now. I'm acting again and attending mass every Sunday. One of my prayers is that my family never has to go through that again. I pray that I may die quickly from anything other than Alzheimer's.

Mine Is "The Family Next Door"

By Meryl Comer, president and CEO of the
Geoffrey Beene Foundation Alzheimer's Initiative

I'm a former TV journalist, not a scientist or a neurologist or a gerontologist. My personal observations would never make it into a medical journal. Let's just say I have put in more than a decade of on-the-job training in the trenches with Alzheimer's disease. While the scientists and doctors are working away in laboratories and clinics, searching for new Alzheimer therapies and protocols, I am at the patient's bedside, trying to deal with the cruel realities of a disease for which there is currently no cure.

My 58-year-old husband was diagnosed with Alzheimer's just 12 years into our marriage. A hematologist/oncologist, he devoted his life's work to unraveling rare blood diseases, never realizing he would be taken down by an incurable disease himself.

The Academy of Neurology reports that pressures on family life start long before active dementia is apparent. There is a distinctive personality profile that seems to be associated with later development of the disease. The person displays increasing inflexibility, self-centeredness and something called "neuroticism," which to the unsuspecting ranks right up there with the garden-variety grounds for divorce.

And then, in our case, the inappropriate and erratic behaviors slowly and progressively got worse. Notes from my journal:

"The hospital doors lock behind us. The man who has been my constant shadow will have to remain sequestered in a special ward for further evaluation. Just two weeks ago, a top neuro doc somehow gave him a clean bill of health. All the trial-and-error protocols with antipsychotics make him more aggressive. He paces the ward, refusing to sit down. I follow and feed him while he walks the halls. Every attempt at personal hygiene is a confrontation. It takes four nurses to hold him still for a blood draw. I have been on the front lines of his daily care, but now I am ignored and dismissed by staff physicians."

Two-and-a-half months later, the doctor's final report and recommendation came: "Diagnosis: Early-onset Alzheimer's with a behavior disorder. Your husband is too dangerous to come home."

The truth is my husband's furies had almost driven me to leave him. But the Alzheimer diagnosis took that escape away by redefining "irreconcilable domestic differences" as a pathology I chose not to walk away from. Did I have a choice? Not in my mind, as a responsible and caring spouse.

I took him home because no facility would have us. Sixteen years later, defying every doctor's prognosis, he is still lingering there in the end stages of Alzheimer's and under my 24/7 care. Here is a snapshot from my night shift:

"I slip between the bedcovers, careful not to disturb the stranger lying there. His eyes are closed, but I take no chances. He is aware of me, but does not know me. I turn into him and begin to breathe in a slow, steady rhythm that mesmerizes him into a temporary slumber. I have learned to succeed where drugs have failed. But the reprieve will be short and the night long. Soon he will wake screaming and flailing his arms, as if fighting off demons. I am his captive, victim to a once-brilliant, but now demented mind. Challenging his outbursts is self-defeating and useless. I play to his realities in order to survive. The terror of his world is my world."

There is another ironic twist to my reality. My 85-year-old mother is battling the disease, too, and lives with us. Of course, she doesn't know it—because the denial that is the gift of Alzheimer's keeps her unaware of what's happening to her, as it did my husband. As her only remaining child, I am now also the target for her rage and paranoia. Misplaced items are now "stolen." Food in the refrigerator is now "poison."

So I am now twice captive to the painful and protracted nightmare I share with millions of baby boomers watching a loved one succumb to Alzheimer's—a cruel disease that is our fate, too, if a cure is not found. For now, it's my lonely destiny to walk ahead of my generation to the dark side of the longevity—but not by much. By the middle of this century, I believe my family will look like "the family next door."

We must mobilize and push for a national research commitment to end Alzheimer's that matches the magnitude of this disease. We must do whatever it takes to make sure ours is the last generation of caregivers with the terrible Hobson's choice—to care or not to care—the last generation trapped by a diagnosis that destroys more lives than just the one of the person who has it. I am terrified for all of us, and time is running out.

Complications: Blended Family Values

By Anonymous, a daughter/stepdaughter living in the Midwest

Alzheimer's is a complicated disease even in the best of circumstances—the best of circumstances being a cohesive, functioning family with enough resources to provide the necessary care.

It's complicated, because Alzheimer's is truly a family disease. It affects every member—emotionally, physically, financially, psychologically. When a family member is stricken with this cruel disease, there is a continual stream of decisions to be made. What doctor to choose? How and when should you tell the patient, family and friends? How to find care? How many times can the person with the disease get lost while driving before you need to take away the driver's license? When and where do you move the family member once he or she can no longer live at home? How to pay for it all?

The decision-making can be a minefield, and the burden of the process can either pull a family together or pull it apart. Complicated, indeed.

But my story takes "complicated" to a whole new level. Ours is a "blended family"—two stepparents, 12 stepchildren, all spread out around the United States.

My mother was only 39 when my father died, leaving her with eight kids. I was the youngest. Mom strengthened herself with her faith and dedicated the next 20 years to raising her family in Chicago. My grandfather would come up from Albuquerque, New Mexico, in the summers to provide a father figure for the kids and moral support for Mom.

After I was grown up and married, my mother went home to New Mexico for a cousin's wedding. She met and started dating George, an old acquaintance. They've been married for 20 years, having had a full life of crafts fairs, sporting events, volunteer work, travel, old friends and new. But now age has caught up with them, and this is where the complications really kick in.

Mom has Alzheimer's. All of her children work and live with their families in the Midwest. But Mom and George—who is in poor health himself—live in New Mexico, where two of his four grown kids are. So that's what we face: two aging parents, one with Alzheimer's, 12 children. Two separate families who barely know each other and myriad decisions.

Although Mom can still clearly state what she wants, she is incapable of recognizing the change in her own abilities and the frailty of her husband's health. She no longer has the reasoning skills to negotiate the decision-making process. So when it's time to figure out health care and doctors, living conditions and finances, Mom is out of the loop. George, worn down by the process, is deferring many of the decisions to his own daughters living locally. Bottom line: George's children are in a position to make many decisions that affect our mother's life.

We know we're fortunate that some of George's family live close by and can help, but this is our mother. Yes, we seem to all get along and want what is best for our parents—for their safety, health and comfort. But there are many ways to reach these goals. How do you decide?

We're a large, extended family with little in common other than our parents' marriage. Our different life experiences create 12 sets of opinions on everything. We're protective of our individual parent's needs, and yet we're conscious that they're a union and need to be respected as such.

So how do you create a flow of information and establish a process for making decisions? Does each family pick a spokesman? Is it the eldest? Or it is the ones who are most involved in the day-to-day issues of care? The truth is, it's one of George's daughters who goes by weekly to help pay bills, schedule doctors appointments and monitor the medicines. And it's usually my sisters or I who field panicked calls from New Mexico about safety or illness.

Recently, we had our first conference call with both families and Mom's doctor. At times it was awkward, but it went OK. It's the best we can do since we live all over the country.

Trusting your mother's care to anyone else is not an easy thing to do, especially with such a complicated and demanding disease as Alzheimer's. But for the moment, I'm staying open-minded. I'm hoping solutions will come through communication. For now, I pray that it's enough.

Women and Alzheimer's in Ethnic Communities

By Gwen Yeo, Ph.D., co-director of the Stanford Geriatric Education Center and fellow of the American Geriatrics Society

*W*hen we're talking about Alzheimer's and women, then we also must talk about Alzheimer's and women from diverse ethnic backgrounds. It's important because ethnic minorities are projected to comprise over 40 percent of all older Americans by 2050, and the majority of these will be women.

Women in general are at greater risk for Alzheimer's than men, but women from some cultural backgrounds bear additional burdens. Whether they're the people with Alzheimer's and other dementing conditions themselves or the caregivers of family members with those diseases, ethnic women's lives are very often heavily impacted by cultural expectations around caregiving.

> *“ In some cultures, there's such a strong expectation that the sick and dying will be cared for at home by family members that outside services and support aren't accessed at all. ”*

In some cultures, there is such a strong expectation that the sick and dying will be cared for at home by family members, that outside services and support aren't accessed at all. The increased burden means women caregivers in these traditions are at even higher risk than other women for the extreme stress, burnout and resulting health effects caregivers are known to suffer.

Here's a brief overview of what we know about people in specific ethnic populations who have Alzheimer's or are Alzheimer caregivers in the United States:

- **African-Americans.** Most studies find that African-Americans have higher rates of vascular dementia resulting from small strokes related to high blood pressure. Some studies have also found higher rates of Alzheimer's disease. These higher rates have been found to be partially explained by the higher incidence of Alzheimer's among elders with low education and low literacy levels, which are common among older African-Americans because of the discrimination many experienced as children. On the caregiving front, the African-American women caring for family elders with dementia may be not just daughters or wives but also nieces, granddaughters or even close friends of the elders. Despite often having fewer resources and having to deal with a higher incidence of behavioral problems among elders with dementia, African-American women have a more positive view of caregiving than others do. They report less depression and less experience of caregiver burden than other groups. They frequently use religion and sometimes humor as coping strategies.

- **American Indian and Alaska Natives.** Unfortunately, there are no comprehensive studies of the risk of Alzheimer's among American Indian or Alaska Native elders in the more than 500 tribes and villages scattered throughout the United States, but there are some tantalizing suggestions that their genetic risk may be lower. On the caregiving side, a study of Pueblo Indian wives and daughters providing care to cognitively impaired elders found that they experienced caregiving as a very heavy burden, with very few or no support services available to them. A primary coping strategy was "passive forbearance"—just accepting and adapting to their situation.

- **Asian-Americans.** There are no studies of the prevalence of Alzheimer's among women in different Asian-American populations, except among Japanese Americans, who were found to have rates in the same range as the majority population, with women's rate slightly higher than men's.

The difference comes in caregiving. In families from most Asian backgrounds, there is an especially strong expectation and obligation to care for one's parents without outside help because of the traditional Asian values of filial piety and family care. Meeting those obligations in the United States, however, is frequently very stressful because adult daughters and daughters-in-law here often work outside the home, and there are few extended family members to share the care as there might have been in the countries of origin. Asian sons sometimes are expected to take on the responsibility of caring for dependent parents, but in reality that frequently means that the son makes the caregiving decisions, while his wife carries the burden of hands-on care. There is an especially strong stigma related to having Alzheimer's in some Asian-American communities, which is a barrier to seeking and receiving assessment and treatment.

- **Latino-Americans.** Studies of the prevalence of Alzheimer's disease among the populations classified as Hispanic or Latino in the United States have shown vastly differing results. A well-known New York study of predominantly Dominican and Puerto Rican elders found much higher rates of Alzheimer's than in the majority population, but a California study among predominantly Mexican-Americans showed rates similar to those found in the majority population. Both of these study populations included large numbers of elders with very little education. Other important findings include the higher risk of dementia among Latino elders with lower folate levels, those with abdominal fat and those with diabetes. This is important because older Latinas have twice the rates of diabetes of older non-Latina white women.

  Latinos were found to have earlier onset of symptoms, more behavioral problems and possibly longer survival, which taken together indicate a much greater burden for their caregivers. In Latino communities, daughters are found to be the most common caregivers, and in spite of the stereotype of large Latino families, many times there are not many other family members sharing responsibility with the designated daughter. The caregivers are more likely to be depressed but less likely to express burden, and they frequently feel under strong cultural obligations to care for parents at home without using outside help.

It's clear that women struggling to cope with dementia of their own or their loved ones in the various ethnic minority populations for which we have information have both unique challenges and unique strengths. Much more information is needed to understand their situations, especially among those populations where data are completely missing.

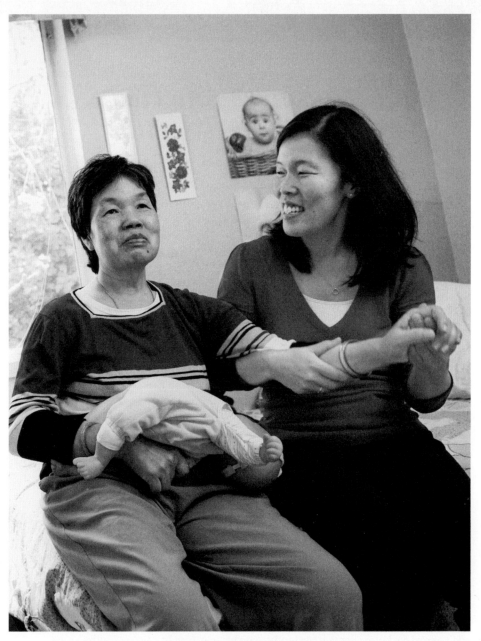

My Quach with her daughter Xuan.

A Vietnamese-American Family Pulls Together

By Xuan Quach, assistant director of the Rotary Center for International Studies in Peace and Conflict Resolution at the University of California, Berkeley

Growing up, I remember my mother coming home from work early each morning, waking us up and helping my younger brother, sisters and me get ready for school. In spite of how tired she was from working all night assembling computer chips at a local factory, my mother always took care of us. She was there when we left for school in the morning, and she was there for us when we came home. She endured long working hours to provide for our family and often worked the hours that no one else wanted, so she could be at home when we were home.

Seven years ago, when she was 56, my mother was diagnosed with younger-onset Alzheimer's disease. Our lives were turned upside down. But in the midst of it all, we knew that as a family we wanted to be involved. We wanted to make sure that Mom was taken care of. Since we were told that there could be a more rapid progression of the disease for those with younger-onset Alzheimer's, we wanted to be there for her right from the beginning—to help take care of our mother in the same way that she took care of all of us.

> **" We wanted to be there for her right from the beginning—to help take care of our mother in the same way that she took care of all of us. "**

At the time, all of us siblings were living in different parts of the world, but Mom's illness brought us back home to Northern California. My sister left her job in New York City, and I moved back from abroad. My brother and his wife bought a house nearby, so we could all live together and look after Mom.

All this happened with much compromise, sacrifice and adjustment on all of our parts. It definitely hasn't been easy. To some degree, we've all put our own agendas on hold, as we've rearranged our lives and schedules around Mom and her care needs. She has become our priority.

> ❝ *We've all put our own agendas on hold, as we've rearranged our lives and schedules around Mom and her care needs. She has become our priority.* ❞

Since her diagnosis, my mother has steadily progressed and is no longer able to carry out simple tasks, such as washing dishes or putting on her own shoes. Eventually, the daily task of caring for her became too much, and we had to make the heart-wrenching decision to place her in a long-term care facility. Up to now, we have all chipped in to help provide for her. But I worry when we will no longer be able to financially support my mother and her long-term care needs. What do we do then? Who will take care of Mom then?

These are the kinds of constant worries that come with taking care of my mother—in addition to watching and worrying about the continuing changes caused by the progression of her disease. Recently, she has started using a cane to walk, and I find it hard to imagine the day when she will no longer be able to walk at all, feed herself or even recognize who I am. Yet I know that such a day will come.

Given all the uncertainties that go along with this devastating disease, when I am with my mother, I have tried to focus on the present moment and simply enjoy the time we have together. Although Alzheimer's has robbed my mother of much of her memory and her ability to communicate with us, it has not taken away her sense of humor, her joy when she hears music and laughter, or her pure happiness when she sees a baby on the street. These moments can still make her laugh and smile. And sometimes, when she's in the mood, she even sings and dances a bit. These are all the moments I treasure, the moments I'll remember, as I continue on this terrible journey called Alzheimer's disease.

The Prescription for a Crisis

By Janet Murguia, president and CEO of the National Council of La Raza

Because the Latino population skews so young, the challenges facing the elderly in our community too often aren't given the attention they deserve. In addition, the Hispanic community faces crisis levels of diabetes, cancer and heart disease, so diseases that affect the mind often aren't part of the discussion.

But make no mistake about it: Alzheimer's and other dementias have had a profound and growing effect on Latinos in this country. There are nearly a 250,000 Latinos suffering from Alzheimer's, and that number is expected to grow 600 percent by the year 2050. And because there is such a high incidence of possible Alzheimer risk factors like diabetes and vascular disease among Hispanics, they are also likely to be diagnosed with Alzheimer's at an earlier age.

> *66 Because there is such a high incidence of possible Alzheimer risk factors like diabetes and vascular disease among Hispanics, they're also likely to be diagnosed with Alzheimer's at an earlier age. 99*

Now add this: The formidable care requirements of Alzheimer's are made more daunting by the Latino community's lower average levels of income and wealth, the lack of access to quality health care and the lack of culturally appropriate Alzheimer literature and programs. Taking all of it together, you have the prescription for a crisis.

These are not just statistics and facts to me.

The most amazing woman I have ever known was diagnosed with Alzheimer's in 2002. Born in a tiny town in Mexico, she emigrated with her husband to the United States nearly 60 years ago, with little money or education to their name. Not only did she do a remarkable job of raising seven children on her husband's factory-worker salary, she added to the family income by caring for many of the other children in her Kansas City, Kansas, neighborhood.

Her devotion and hard work bore fruit. Over the years, she celebrated her son's and grandson's graduations from Ivy League law schools, saw her daughter and son become federal judges and visited her daughter's office in the West Wing of the White House. Her hard work, faith, wisdom and kindness are the stuff of legend in the Argentine section of Kansas City.

That woman's name is Amalia Murguia, and she is my mother.

My brothers, sisters and I are fortunate that we have the resources and access to good health care to help our mother in her battle with Alzheimer's. We are lucky there are so many of us to share the burden and that she has the very best possible caregiver in my sister Rose Mary. But all of us who love her know firsthand the toll—the physical, financial and, most of all, emotional toll—of seeing this horrible disease slowly rob us of the mother, grandmother, neighbor and friend we cherish and revere. And the burden is especially acute for primary caregivers, who will play an increasingly critical role as we battle Alzheimer's in the future.

I am trying to make peace with the fact that the best my family can do for the foreseeable future is make my mom's life as comfortable as possible. But I have not made peace with the notion that there is nothing I can do to fight this enemy.

I am very proud that my organization, the National Council of La Raza, established one of the first Alzheimer projects targeting the Latino population. I am working to raise awareness and bring attention to the effects Alzheimer's has on our community.

I will not rest until we have a better way to cope with this disease and, perhaps, even a cure. I owe it to my mom and to all the other beloved moms and dads out there—and to their families.

A Couple Copes

By Jill Eikenberry and Michael Tucker, award-winning Broadway,
TV and film actors best known for their roles in the hit TV drama L.A. Law.
They've been married 37 years.

Jill's Story

Everything was wonderful. My husband, Mike, and I were enjoying a lovely semi-retirement, living in New York and Italy. My mom, Lora, was living with her second husband in a beautiful retirement community in Santa Barbara, where I was sure they would live out their last years.

But then my mother's husband died, and it became clear she was declining mentally. It was difficult for me to admit, but she was in a lot worse shape than I'd thought. Her husband had apparently been covering for her for years. When she hit her head in a couple of falls, things went even further downhill—fast. I felt I had no choice but to bring her to New York to live near us.

Mike was very resistant because he thought it would impact our beautiful life, and of course he was right. But what could I do? I'm an only child, and my mother had always needed me. When she was 32, she had developed a severe hearing loss, and I began to translate the world for her. I've always felt I was the only one who could save my mother.

Moving Mom created its own set of problems. We had her in an assisted care facility three blocks away. Now, in addition to being widowed and suffering several hits on the head, she was in an unfamiliar place. She was very resistant to having round-the-clock aides, but she needed them. When a caregiver didn't know how to put her hearing aid in, I would run over and demonstrate, but the next day a different helper would show up, and she wouldn't know how to do it, either. When Mom couldn't hear the aide coming up behind her to help put a sweater on or dry her off after the shower, she became belligerent. She would often take a swing at the caregivers and sometimes even connect. Mom was getting a terrible reputation in the facility. Nobody wanted to work with her.

Every day I went to the woman in charge and screamed that half their patients had some form of dementia and they just had to find aides who knew how to deal with it. But even when we would get a good caregiver, the facility wouldn't assign her to Mom on a regular basis.

So when an apartment became available across the hall from ours, we took it. What else could we do? Now it meant that I was the one who had to find the right caregivers—but I didn't know how to run a nursing home! How would I be able to trust someone just on the basis of one interview?

Just when I was about to lose hope, in walked Marcia—the tall, beautiful, kind and loving Jamaican woman who has changed our lives.

Marcia "got" my mother immediately, and she taught me a huge lesson. She made my mom laugh. I saw that Marcia didn't need my mother to be the intellectual and the political activist she'd always been. She fell in love with the person my mother had become. She even renamed her—she calls her Lolo. And Marcia's acceptance of my mother just the way she is has helped not only me, but also Mom herself, to relax—to stop trying to hold on to the person she could no longer be.

My mother was never affectionate. Because of the hearing loss, she always talked a lot, rarely about personal things—throwing out a wall of words to fill up the spaces when she couldn't hear. She did that with me, too. But now I have a completely new relationship with her, and in some ways it's quite wonderful. Since she has aphasia, she can say only a few words at a time, and most of the time she doesn't bother. She gives me a warm smile when I walk into the room. She holds out her arms to me, we have a long hug, and then we sit on the couch and hold hands.

A very long time ago, I said to Mike that I just wanted a few moments with my mom when we could just sit together and hold hands and not talk. Now I have that every day.

Mike's Take

When Jill and I bought our little farmhouse in Italy almost seven years ago, we thought we were blithely setting off on a romantic idyll, eager to explore the next chapter of our lives. Our kids were out in the world—Alison with a successful career as a private chef in Los Angeles and Max an up-and-coming drummer on the New York music scene. Our only living parent—Jill's mom, Lora—was living well with her husband in Santa Barbara. "Everyone's settled," we thought. "Off we go!"

Well, not so fast, Buster. After her husband died, Lora—an energetic, independent and fiercely intellectual 86-year-old—began to show signs of advancing dementia. Jill said there was nothing to do but move her mom closer to us. We were her only family.

Bye-bye, romantic retirement.

Now, it's true I had always had a difficult time warming up to Lora, but before you call me the bad guy, know that I agreed that we should move her across the country to New York. That made sense. Plus, I couldn't very well play the part of the unfeeling, self-serving son-in-law. That kind of role can end a career. But I did see that scary look in Jill's eyes— the look of a savior, the gleam of missionary zeal—and I was terrified that retirement life as we knew it, as we had brilliantly created it, was in peril.

I'd seen it happen before. We know a couple who decided to put off their own retirement dreams until after her mother, an 87-year-old with advanced cancer, passed on. Well, the mother lived 12 more long years, and by the time she died, our friends were too old to do anything more strenuous than oatmeal. I was adamant that in our family, we'd find a way to both take care of Lora and also have our beautiful retirement together at the same time.

But in the middle of all this, other changes started to occur. Alison decided to move back to New York, where she had grown up. She and her brother Max, who'd never lived in the same city since childhood, found an apartment together, just up Broadway from where we live.

Suddenly and miraculously and remarkably and for the first time, our family—which had always been a loose network of individual strands—became a functioning unit. And it remains so today.

Alison's first job as a private chef in New York was to cook all the meals for her grandmother, who, by that time, was living with caregivers across the hall from us. We all look out for each other's security and well-being, cover for each other, even feed each other. I'm amazed that the key to pulling all of us together is not only Lora, my mother-in-law, but also Alison, Jill's stepdaughter. It's so extraordinary, I sometimes have to pinch myself. We're a family. It's all very Italian.

66 Suddenly and miraculously and remarkably and for the first time, our family—which had always been a loose network of individual strands—became a functioning unit. And it remains so today. 99

Which brings us to the other major character in the story—Italy itself. Our time there helped produce our transformation. In America, the accepted wisdom is that we don't bring our aged parents home, we find a place for them to go to. The Italians, conversely, make a place for them at home. We didn't realize we were being moved in this direction, but looking back, there's no question that our new family template is modeled on what we saw around us in Italy.

Our experience, which started out so traumatically, turned out to be a true journey home. It's about children becoming adults right before our eyes. It's about an aged parent becoming a child. It's about Jill and I realizing once again that the direction our life takes isn't the issue—it only matters that we're moving in that direction together.

Are We Prepared?

Is America Ready for the Economic Impact of Alzheimer's?

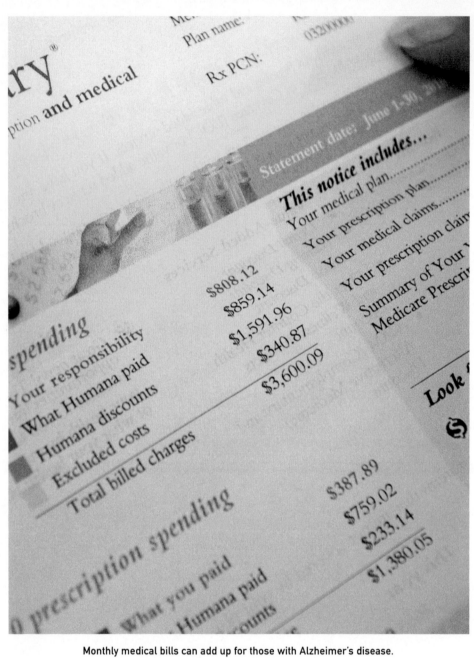

Monthly medical bills can add up for those with Alzheimer's disease.

The Cost of Alzheimer's

"When Alzheimer's first invaded our lives, we were so thankful that we had three sources of medical insurance. Now our whole financial world is in ruins, and it's down to just Medicare."

"I sometimes wish there were a different way to care for my mother—one that doesn't cost me work time and wages to be with her."

"How can I increase my earnings, when I can't do the job I know I would do if I didn't have Alzheimer's putting roadblocks in my way?"

"I wish I didn't have to turn down job opportunities in other parts of the country because I can't imagine asking my husband to leave his mother when she needs him the most."

"I worry when we will no longer be able to financially support my mother and her long-term care needs. What do we do then? Who will take care of Mom then?"

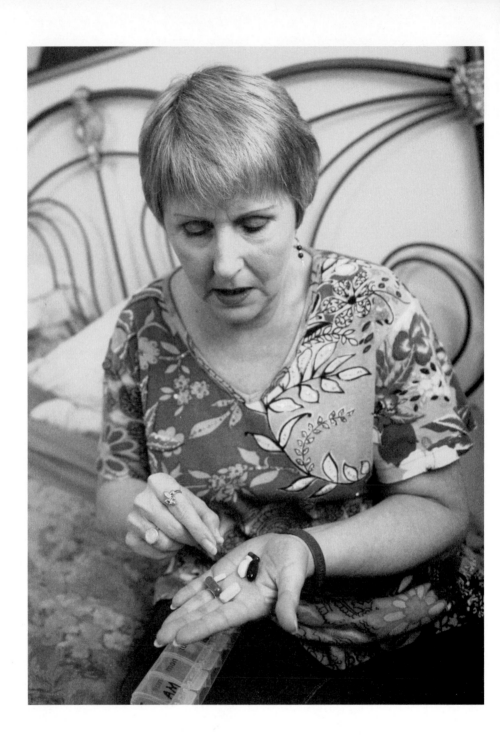

Is America Ready for the Economic Impact of Alzheimer's?

By Brent D. Fulton, Ph.D.

I n analysis of prior cost-of-illness studies reveals the economic cost of Alzheimer's disease to be an estimated $300 billion a year, projected to double or triple by 2050. The cost per person with Alzheimer's is about $56,800 annually, and families bear three-fifths of these costs to the tune of some $34,500, mostly from providing unpaid caregiving services.

But while the numbers are huge, they don't begin to describe in personal terms the financial toll, not to mention the enormous mental, emotional and physical hardship on caregivers, especially women.

Consider the McCormacks:

When Patricia McCormack's mother, Helen, called unusually early one morning and began asking where Patricia lived, alarm bells went off. Both Patricia and her grown daughter, Seraphina Uludong, flew from the West Coast to Buffalo, New York, to check on Helen. The pair soon realized Helen likely had Alzheimer's disease and would no longer be able to live independently. They also noticed her home was in disrepair and found many unpaid bills. Thus, a decision was made: Patricia, Seraphina (and her husband, Kenton) would move to Buffalo to care for Helen.

The transition was difficult. Not only was it difficult to witness Helen's decline, Patricia had to sell her home in Portland. And Seraphina, who had been helping her husband with a startup firm, now had to shift her focus to her grandmother's care. She and her mother devoted countless hours over the next three years seeking the appropriate long-term care facilities for Helen. First, she found her a memory-care facility costing $108,000 per year. But then Helen broke her neck and had to be transferred to a rehabilitation facility. Seraphina then found an assisted-living facility that cost $84,000 yearly, but Helen broke her hip and had to be transferred to another rehabilitation facility. After those three years, she found her a nursing home where she currently lives that costs $108,000 per year.

Helen didn't have long-term care insurance, and Medicare only covered her rehabilitation services. Her $30,000 annual income wasn't enough to cover long-term care in a nursing home. And she didn't initially qualify for Medicaid because she had $60,000 in savings, though it was depleted in less than two years. After that, she had to borrow against her home to pay for long-term care.

Not only were Helen's savings depleted, but Seraphina's and Kenton's savings shrunk, too, as they paid $15,000 for some of Helen's care and their own moving expenses. And while it's difficult to put a price on Seraphina's time away from the business, clearly it would run into the tens of thousands of dollars. Patricia incurred numerous expenses from selling her home to move across the country.

What's more, the entire family's healthcare needs and costs increased. Patricia's out-of-pocket healthcare costs increased because caregiving stress contributed to her illnesses. Seraphina, for the first time, suffered panic attacks from the stress of managing Helen's care. Her own health insurance lapsed, and she couldn't afford New York's relatively higher premiums for young adults. Being uninsured added to her stress.

Life has begun to calm down a bit for the McCormacks. Helen is stable in a nursing home and was finally able to qualify for Medicaid after five years. The family is trying to sell her home. They all moved back to the West Coast and are rebuilding their savings, and Seraphina and Kenton are growing their business.

As the McCormacks' story shows, discovering that a family member has Alzheimer's can mark the beginning of a brutal period for everyone, not only emotionally but financially. Of the approximate annual $300 billion cost of Alzheimer's in the United States, families bear much of this financial cost and risk, including almost $150 billion for informal, unpaid care provided by themselves and friends.

Medicare does not cover long-term care, and only 7 million people in the United States have long-term care insurance. Medicaid is designed to cover long-term care for the poor, but it requires families to spend down their assets to become eligible. To mitigate some of this financial risk, a national voluntary long-term insurance plan will be created under the Community Living Assistance Services and Supports (CLASS) Act, which was part of the recently passed healthcare reform.

This chapter provides estimates of the current and projected costs of Alzheimer's disease, examines how those costs are financed and discusses policy options aimed at mitigating the disease's economic impact on the country and families.

Economic cost of Alzheimer's disease

The economic cost of Alzheimer's disease impacts both people with Alzheimer's and caregivers. Patient care includes long-term care and health care, and caregivers require additional health care because of the stress of caregiving.

Medicare does not cover long-term care,
and only 7 million people in the United States
have long-term care insurance.

Long-term care includes personal care services, such as helping people with activities of daily living (ADL)—like eating, dressing, bathing, using the toilet and getting in and out of bed. It also includes instrumental activities of daily living (IADL), such as light household chores, managing money, shopping and taking medications. These personal care services may be provided in the community or at a facility. Approximately 70 percent of people with Alzheimer's reside in the community,[1] which is typically the person's or a relative's home, and may be augmented with local adult daycare and professional home health aides. Most of the care is provided by unpaid family and friends. Because these services are not purchased in the market, they are considered informal care. Facility-based care typically occurs in a nursing home.

In addition to long-term care, people with Alzheimer's require health care, including Alzheimer's disease diagnostic services, medications to treat symptoms and treatment for co-morbidities, which may be exacerbated by Alzheimer's disease.

Alzheimer's does not just affect the individual with the disease. Caregivers require more health care as a result of caregiving. Several studies have shown that caregivers report increased stress as a result of caregiving.[2] Women disproportionately bear this stress and its cost. The Alzheimer's Association Women and Alzheimer's poll found that approximately 60 percent of unpaid caregivers for people with Alzheimer's disease or other dementias were women.[3] Of those women, 68 percent reported emotional stress as a result of caregiving, and 51 percent acknowledged physical stress. Such stress can negatively impact the caregiver's health and healthcare costs, from increased emergency room visits and hospitalizations[4] to lower life expectancy.[5]

Net patient care costs per individual with Alzheimer's disease

The economic cost of patient care—long-term care and health care—for individuals with Alzheimer's disease has been estimated in several studies, producing a wide range of estimates.[6,7,8,9,10] However, almost all studies point to the high cost of Alzheimer's disease. Broadly speaking, there are two types of economic cost-of-illness studies. Total cost studies estimate the long-term care and healthcare costs for individuals with Alzheimer's disease. The second type—known as excess or net-cost studies—estimates the portion of the total costs that are directly attributable to Alzheimer's disease. These studies compare the costs of individuals with Alzheimer's disease to individuals without Alzheimer's disease and adjust for differences between these two groups based on factors that influence costs, such as age, sex, geographic location and co-morbid conditions. This chapter focuses on net-cost studies, which are the more common type, because they can be used to estimate savings from slowing the progression of the disease to finding a cure.

Based on the studies presented in Table 2, which were inflated to 2010 dollars, the estimated annual net cost of patient care is $50,200 for people with Alzheimer's residing in the community and $69,400 for those residing in facilities. Based on 70 percent of people with Alzheimer's residing in the community,[10] then the average cost per patient for patient care is $56,000. This estimate is consistent with Ernst & Hay,[11] which reviewed previous studies and estimated annual net costs to be $53,500.

> Unpaid family caregivers spend $4 billion a year on their own health care due to the stress and strain of caregiving.

The $56,000 estimate includes $28,800 for care that is purchased in the market, such as nursing home care, adult daycare services and health care. This care is referred to as formal care. In contrast, the remaining $27,200 in costs is for care that is not purchased in the market, but instead includes unpaid services—primarily caregiving services—provided by family and friends. This care is referred to as informal care. As expected, the informal care costs are significantly higher in the community versus a facility, because community care is often provided by unpaid family members, particularly women. Not surprisingly, over half (56 percent) of the Alzheimer caregivers surveyed in the Alzheimer's Association Women and Alzheimer's poll reported a significant strain on their family's finances as a result of their caregiving.[3]

The informal care cost estimates are usually based on the cost to hire a home health aide, not the wages that the unpaid caregiver could have earned in the labor market if he or she was not providing care. This is because home health aide wage data are readily available, and it is difficult to estimate the wages of individuals who are not in the labor force, particularly retired persons providing unpaid care.

With 5.3 million individuals in the United States suffering from Alzheimer's disease, the annual net cost to the country is $301 billion.

However, some caregivers providing informal care are also employed. According to the 2010 Families and Work Institute Study on Eldercare, two in five employed individuals have provided elder care within the past five years.[12] Of those who provided caregiving, 38 percent reported taking time off work or cutting back on work hours to allow more time for caregiving, and one-half of these individuals reported losing income.

Increased health care costs per caregiver

Few studies have estimated unpaid caregivers' increased healthcare costs as a result of the stress associated with caregiving. A survey of 17,000 employees of a multinational firm based in the United States estimated that caregivers' healthcare costs were 8 percent higher than non-caregivers', a difference of approximately $530 per year.[13,14] A study from the early 1990s estimated the costs to be $350 per year (adjusted to 2010 dollars using medical care inflation).[11] The $530 estimate is likely to be a conservative estimate, because caregiving for people with Alzheimer's is more stressful than caregiving for most people who don't have the disease.

Net cost of Alzheimer's disease in the United States

Table 1 presents the annual net-cost estimates per individual with Alzheimer's disease previously discussed and aggregates these costs for the entire United States for 2010. The annual net cost per person with Alzheimer's is $56,800. Based on 5.3 million individuals in the United States having Alzheimer's disease,[15,16] the annual net cost to the country is $301 billion. This cost estimate is based on the best available studies;

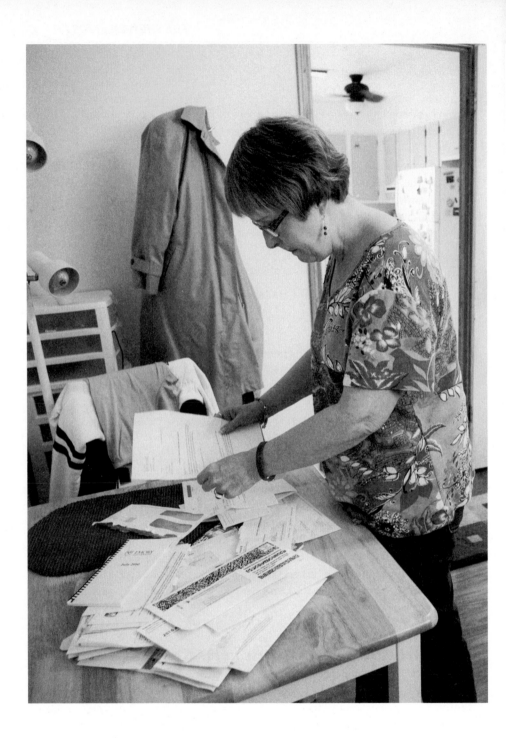

TABLE 1 : Annual Net Cost Estimates for Alzheimer's
Disease in the United States, 2010

Cost Categories	Costs ($ 2010)
Cost Per Patient	
Patient's long-term care and healthcare costs	$28,800
Patient's unpaid caregiving costs provided by family and friends	$27,200
Caregiver's increased healthcare costs, as a result of caregiving	$800
Total cost per patient	**$56,800**
Prevalence of Alzheimer's disease (millions)	5.3
Total Cost (billions)	
Patients' long-term care and healthcare costs	$153
Patients' unpaid caregiving costs provided by family and friends	$144
Caregivers' increased healthcare costs, as a result of caregiving	$4
Total cost	**$301**

notwithstanding, cost-of-illness studies have study design and data limitations, so the
approximate $300 billion estimate should not be viewed as exact.

The $56,800 cost per individual with Alzheimer's disease includes $28,000 in long-
term care and healthcare costs, $27,200 in unpaid caregiving costs provided by family
and friends and $800 in caregivers' increased healthcare costs as a result of caregiving[a].
When these costs are aggregated across the estimated 5.3 million individuals with
Alzheimer's disease, the long-term care and healthcare costs are $153 billion, the unpaid
caregiving costs are $144 billion, and the caregivers' increased healthcare costs are
$4 billion, totaling $301 billion.

By 2050, even if the cost per individual with Alzheimer's disease remains the same,[b] the annual cost of Alzheimer's disease in the United States is expected to double or triple, because the disease's prevalence is expected to increase to between 11.5 million and 16.2 million individuals.[15,16]

Financing of Alzheimer's disease costs

Even though the cost of Alzheimer's disease is enormous, families bear most of the costs and financial risk because relatively few have private long-term care insurance. Furthermore, Medicare does not pay for long-term care, and Medicaid only pays for long-term care for the poor, requiring families to spend down their assets in order to become eligible.

Kemper and colleagues (2005) estimated that individuals over 65 will need an average of three years of long-term care, and 20 percent will need more than five years. Because women live longer than men, 28 percent of women will need more than five years of long-term care, while only 11 percent of men will need that amount of care.[17]

This section discusses the major payers of health care and long-term care for individuals with Alzheimer's disease.

Medicare

Medicare pays for healthcare costs associated with Alzheimer's disease, but does not cover long-term care. The major healthcare costs include physician services, hospitalizations and medications. Medicare also covers acute skilled nursing facility care, home health care and hospice care. In the first two cases, personal care services are covered as part of that skilled care, even if the care is provided in a long-term care facility. Medicare covers up to 100 days of skilled nursing facility care if the needed care both follows and is directly related to a hospitalization lasting three or more days. There is no co-payment for days 1 to 20; the co-payment for days 21 to 100 is $137.50 per day in 2010. Skilled nursing facility stays averaged 25 days in 2007.[18]

To qualify for Medicare's home health care, a person must require skilled care, such as care from a skilled nurse or a skilled physical, speech or occupational therapist. In these cases, Medicare will also cover personal care services. There is no limit on the number of visits. In 2004, approximately 6 percent of Medicare beneficiaries used home health services, averaging 31 home health visits.[18]

Hospice care is covered by Medicare for people in the advanced stages of an illness who are expected to live for six months or less. It does not cover personal care services, but does cover respite care for caregivers whereby the patient is transferred to a facility for up to five days.

Medicaid

Medicaid covers long-term care for the poor, and each state has different eligibility requirements based on income or assets.[19] In 2006, Medicaid was the largest payer of long-term care services, paying 40 percent of the $177.6 billion tab. In comparison, Medicare paid 23 percent, which finances skilled care. To be eligible for Medicaid, an elderly individual's income cannot exceed a particular limit, which is often tied to the Supplemental Security Income (SSI) benefit (e.g., up to 300 percent of SSI). In 2010, the SSI benefit is $647 per month for an individual and $1,011 for a family. An individual's assets cannot exceed $2,000, but a home or a spouse's assets can sometimes be protected.

Long-term care insurance

Long-term care insurance is relatively rare, given the financial risk families bear. As of 2008, approximately 7 million adults in the United States had long-term care insurance.[20] This is a low number, considering the number of people who could likely afford to purchase long-term care insurance. Based on a preliminary study, the number of insured represents only 6.4 percent of adults who are not on Medicaid, who would likely pass underwriting standards and whose premium would be less than 7 percent of their income, a proxy for affordability.[20]

Interestingly, in the Alzheimer's Association Women and Alzheimer's poll, nearly a third of men and a quarter of women—representing approximately 66 million adults— reported having long-term care insurance, indicating many Americans believe they have long-term care insurance when they do not. This is because many people erroneously believe that Medicare or their private health insurance covers long-term care.

Summary of financing of Alzheimer's disease costs

Figure 1 shows the financing sources for the cost of Alzheimer's disease, including long-term care and health care for people with Alzheimer's as well as caregivers' increased healthcare costs. It shows the financing for individuals located in the community and facility settings, as well as the average, based on 70 percent of people with Alzheimer's residing in the community.[c] In community settings, the financing of Alzheimer care is mostly informal care (68 percent) provided by unpaid family and friends.[d] Medicare constitutes the next highest share at 26 percent. In facility settings, the respective shares of Medicaid (29 percent), out of pocket (29 percent) and Medicare (26 percent) are similar;

informal care is only 13 percent and private insurance is only 0.8 percent. In facilities, Medicare is typically financing short-term skilled care, followed by a family's out-of-pocket expenditures until assets are spent down to qualify for Medicaid.[21]

Based on the mix of financing between community and facility settings—the "Average" column in Figure 1—and that the net cost of Alzheimer's disease is $56,800 per patient yearly, families bear $34,500, or three-fifths of the costs. This burden is nearly the annual cost of attending a private four-year university, estimated to be $39,000 for the 2009-2010 school year.[22] These costs are a combination of $27,200 for informal care and $7,300 for out-of-pocket expenses. These costs can last several years. Estimates of the median survival after the onset of dementia had varied between five and nine years, but a more recent estimate suggests three years, because it accounted for people with a rapidly progressive illness who died before they would typically be included in a study.[23]

FIGURE 1 : Financing of Alzheimer's Economic Cost in the United States

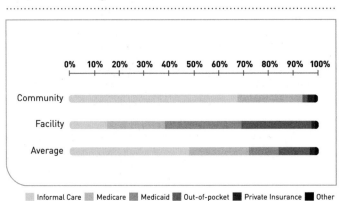

Policy options

With the baby boomer generation reaching 65 and people living longer, Alzheimer's disease is going to become an increasing burden—unless a cure is discovered—on families, particularly women, and society at large. In 2005, there were approximately 37 million individuals aged 65 or older in the United States, representing 12 percent of the population.[24] By 2030, that number is expected to almost double to 70 million, representing 20 percent of the population. Moreover, the number of individuals aged 80 and over is

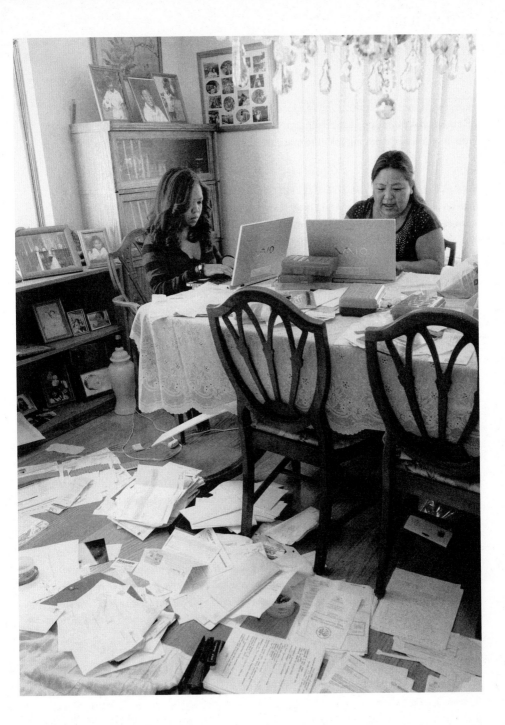

expected to increase from 11 million to 20 million during this same period. This section discusses policy options concerning medical research on Alzheimer's disease, long-term care insurance and paying for informal care.

Medical research on Alzheimer's disease

The level of investment for Alzheimer research is influenced by the disease's health impact, economic cost and the potential for scientific progress toward a cure. Alzheimer research funding competes with other medical research funding, such as cardiovascular disease and cancer, as well as non-medical research. Because of inconclusive evidence, it is beyond the scope of this chapter to estimate the cost effectiveness of current treatments and the amount of funding that should be devoted to Alzheimer research. Instead, it first discusses reviews of cost-effectiveness studies of current treatments. Second, it discuss overall medical research funding in the United States and the criteria that shapes the National Institutes of Health's (NIH) research-funding decisions.

The goal of the research is to find a cure for Alzheimer's disease. Short of that, research is ongoing to better diagnose patients in the hopes that treatments will be more effective if Alzheimer's is diagnosed early. In addition, research exists to develop treatments to improve mental functioning of individuals with Alzheimer's disease. Currently, a diagnosis is made based on symptoms because a definitive diagnosis can only be made by examining a person's brain after death. New technologies are being developed to identify the presence of the disease before symptoms become apparent, in the hopes that eventual treatments will be more successful if Alzheimer's disease is detected early.[25]

Five medications are approved by the U.S. Food and Drug Administration to improve the mental functioning of individuals with Alzheimer's disease, allowing them to perform more activities of daily living, which temporarily reduces caregiver costs.[26,27] However, the medications' effects are temporary and become less effective as the disease progresses. The cost-effectiveness studies have been inconclusive because of the difficulty of measuring the quality of life of people with Alzheimer's disease as well as the various methods used to estimate costs.[28,29,30]

With respect to future treatments, Murphy and Topel argue in their book *Measuring the Gains from Medical Research* that the United States spends too little on medical research in general, given the economic benefits.[31] However, given the uncertainty surrounding medical research and the various ways to measure the burden of a disease, methods are still being developed to determine the optimal amount to be invested for a particular disease. For example, studies usually do not incorporate the disease's burden on caregivers, which is significant for Alzheimer's disease. Moreover, studies usually only consider the benefit of curing a specific disease, even though the cured person's quality of life may not significantly improve because he or she is then afflicted with another disease, such as Alzheimer's, because of its increased risk as a person ages.

In 2007, biomedical research totaled $101.1 billion (approximately 5 percent of healthcare expenditures), including $27.8 billion from the NIH, $36.6 billion from pharmaceutical firms and $15.3 billion from biotechnology firms.[32] For Alzheimer's disease, there were no readily available estimates of public and private research funding. For example, the NIH funding for Alzheimer research in fiscal year 2009 (October 1, 2008, to September 30, 2009) totaled $534 million, including $77 million from the American Recovery & Reinvestment Act.[33] However, additional NIH funds for Alzheimer research are included in more general categories such as clinical trials and neuroscience.

The NIH Working Group on Priority Setting listed the following five general criteria that shape NIH's funding decisions: (1) public health needs, (2) scientific quality of the research, (3) potential for basic scientific progress, (4), portfolio diversification and (5) and support human and physical capital.[34] Alzheimer's disease is a significant public health need and will become increasingly so with the aging population. Among a number of bills, the Alzheimer's Association is advocating for the passage of the Alzheimer's Breakthrough Act, which would authorize $2 billion per year for Alzheimer research at the NIH.[35] This funding level would still be well below NIH's fiscal year 2009 budgets for genetics ($9 billion) and cancer ($6.7 billion) research.[33]

Long-term care insurance and the CLASS Act

Families face financial uncertainty given the potential costs of long-term care associated with Alzheimer's disease. Medicare does not cover long-term care, and the private long-term care insurance market only covers 7 million individuals. Although Medicaid provides a safety net, families are not eligible until they spend down their assets.

To mitigate some of this financial risk, the Community Living Assistance Services and Supports (CLASS) Act was signed into law as part of the Patient Protection and Affordable Care Act (PPACA), the healthcare reform passed in March 2010. The CLASS Act creates a national voluntary long-term care federal insurance program for adults.[36,37]

The program began January 1, 2011, and is administered by the U.S. Department of Health and Human Services. It is financed by individuals' premiums through payroll deductions of participating employers. Self-employed individuals or employees working for non-participating employers are able to enroll through an alternative mechanism. Because the program is voluntary, employees can opt out.

An individual becomes vested after paying five years of premiums. Premiums are age-adjusted, and the premium level is set so that the program remains solvent for 75 years. Benefit levels are based on the degree of disability or impairment, and the level is at least $50 per day and is expected to average approximately $75 per day. There is no lifetime benefit cap. A vested individual who is currently paying premiums becomes eligible for benefits if he or she cannot perform two or more activities of daily living or has an equivalent cognitive disability, such as Alzheimer's disease.

Because of the current recession, at least 25 states and Washington, D.C., have either cut long-term care services or significantly increased patient cost sharing.

The CLASS program is an important step to reduce the families' financial risk associated with long-term care. It is not intended to replace Medicaid's long-term care funding or long-term care insurance, but will significantly supplement it. Based on the 2010 Genworth Cost of Care Survey, the median rate for a private nursing home room is $75,190 per year, or $206 per day, much higher than the likely CLASS program benefit.[38] Therefore, to bridge this gap, it is important for policy makers to ensure Medicaid has sufficient financing and that private, long-term care insurance markets operate efficiently.

Paying for informal care

Almost half of the approximate $300 billion annual cost for Alzheimer's disease is supplied by unpaid caregivers. Historically, it is has been controversial whether legally responsible persons—that is, parents of minor children or spouses—should be paid to provide care. However, this is changing. Based on a 2003 survey of caregiver support programs by state, all but six states have at least one program in which relatives may be hired.[39] However, two-thirds of the programs prohibit hiring parents and one-third prohibit hiring spouses.[40]

Because of the current recession, at least 25 states and Washington, D.C., have either cut long-term care services or significantly increased patient cost sharing.[41] For example, Florida has cut Medicaid reimbursements for community-based services for the elderly, such as meals and homemaker services. State Medicaid budget cuts adversely impact adult daycare services, which many Alzheimer families rely on for caregiving respites. These cuts may save money in these states in the short run, but evidence suggests that states with more established home- and community-based services will realize long-term cost savings because of reduced institutional spending.[42]

TABLE 2 : Annual Net Cost Estimates for Patient Care per Individual with Alzheimer's Disease [43,44,45]

Study	Data Years	Sample	Control Group and Method	Formal Costs ($ 2010)	Informal Costs ($ 2010)	Total Costs ($ 2010)
Community						
Bynum (2009)	2004	Medicare Current Beneficiaries Survey, nationally representative sample (n = 16,000) of Medicare population	Non-demented Individuals	$9,700	NA	NA
Langa et al. (2001)	1993	Assets and Health Dynamics Study nationally representative sample (n = 7,443) of community-dwelling individuals aged 70 or older	Non-demented individuals and controlled for sex, age, race, net-worth, co-morbidities	NA	$12,000	NA
Rice et al. (1993)	1988-1990	Sample of individuals (n = 93) with Alzheimer's disease in non-institutionalized settings in Northern California	Caregiver judgement and billing records used to estimate net costs	$21,000	$57,600	$78,600
Average (Community)				**$15,400**	**$34,800**	**$50,200**
Facility						
Bynum (2009)	2004	Medicare Current Beneficiaries Survey, nationally representative sample (n = 16,000) of Medicare population	Non-demented Individuals	$50,000	NA	NA
Rice et al. (1993)	1988-1990	Sample of individuals (n = 94) with Alzheimer's disease in institutionalized settings in Northern California	Caregiver judgement and billing records used to estimate net costs	$70,200	$9,300	$79,500
Average (Facility)				**$60,100**	**$9,300**	**$69,400**
Formal, informal, and total costs (weighted average) (1)				**$28,800**	**$27,200**	**$56,000**

NA: Not applicable because the study did not include this estimate
All dollar amounts are inflated to 2010 dollars
(1) The weighted average is based on 70% of the Alzheimer's patients residing in the community

Table 2 shows the studies used to estimate the annual net patient care costs per individual with Alzheimer's disease within community and facility settings.[e] These studies were based in the United States, used a net-cost approach and had the fewest methodological limitations.[f]

Conclusion

The annual net cost of Alzheimer's disease in the United States is approximately $300 billion, including almost $150 billion for informal, unpaid care provided by family and friends. Women are disproportionately affected because they have a higher Alzheimer's disease prevalence and they are more likely to be caregivers. Policies need to address how to reduce the financial impact of Alzheimer's disease on families. The CLASS Act's national voluntary long-term care insurance program is a start in easing the financial burden and risk on families. But those facing the high costs of nursing home care will remain vulnerable, and the government needs to adopt policies to address this ongoing problem. Further studies need to estimate the appropriate level of public research funding for Alzheimer's disease, given its high prevalence and cost, both of which are expected to grow dramatically because of the aging population.

ENDNOTES

1   Alzheimer's Association, *2010 Alzheimer's Disease Facts and Figures, Alzheimer's and Dementia* 6; 2010a.

2   L. Etters, D. Goodall, B.E. Harrison, "Caregiver burden among dementia patient caregivers: A review of the literature," *Journal of the American Academy of Nurse Practitioners* 20 (2008): 423–428.

3   Alzheimer's Association 2010 Women and Alzheimer's poll.

4   C.C. Schubert, M. Boustani, C.M. Callahan, A.J. Perkins, AJ, S. Hui, H.C. Hendrie, "Acute care utilization by dementia caregivers within urban primary care practices," *Journal of Generai Internal Medicine.* 23.11 (2008): 1736-1740.

5   N.A. Christakis, P.D. Allison, "Mortality after the hospitalization of a spouse," *New England Journal of Medicine.* Vol. 354 (2006): 719-730.

6   W. Quentin, S.G. Riedel-Heller, M. Luppa, A. Rudolph, H.H König, "Cost-of-illness studies of dementia: a systematic review focusing on stage dependency of costs," *ACTA Psychiatrica Scandinavica,* 121;2010: 243-259.

7   B.S. Bloom, N.D. Pouvourville, W.L. Straus, "Cost of Illness of Alzheimer's Disease: How Useful Are Current Estimates?" *The Gerontologist.* 43.2 (2003): 158-164.

8   G.M. Leung, R.Y.T Yeung, I. Chi, L.W. Chu, "The Economics of Alzheimer Disease," *Dementia and Geriatric Cognitive Disorders.* Vol. 13 (2003): 34-43.

9   A. Wimo, G. Ljunggren, B. Winblad, "Costs of Dementia and Dementia Care: A Review." *International Journal of Geriatric Psychiatry* 12;1997: 841-856.

10 R.L. Ernst, J.W. Hay, "Economic Research on Alzheimer Disease: A Review of Literature," *Alzheimer Disease and Associated Disorders.* 11.S6 (1997): 135-145.

11 R.L. Ernst, J.W. Hay, "The US Economic and Social Costs of Alzheimer's Disease Revisited," *American Journal of Public Health.* 84.8 (August 1994): 1261-1264.

12 K. Aumann, E. Galinsky, K. Sakai, M. Brown, J.T. Bond, *Working Family Caregivers of the Elderly: Everyday Realities and Wishes for Change,* New York, NY: Families and Work Institute, 2010.

13 S.M. Albert, R. Schulz, *The MetLife Study of Working Caregivers and Employer Health Care Costs,* New York, NY: MetLife Mature Market Institute, 2010.

14 Centers for Medicare and Medicaid Services, Office of the Actuary, National Health Statistics Group, *Total Personal Health Care Per Capita Spending, By Age Group, Calendar Years, 1987, 1996, 1999, 2002, 2004 and Personal Health Care Spending by Age Group and Source of Payment, Calendar Year 2004, Total Payer (in millions)* https://www.cms.gov/NationalHealthExpendData/downloads/2004-age-tables.pdf, accessed August 18, 2010.

15 L.E. Hebert, P.A. Scherr, J.L. Bienias, D.A. Bennett, D.A. Evans, "Alzheimer Disease in the US Population: Prevalence Estimates Using the 2000 Census," *Archives of Neurology.* Vol. 60 (August 2003): 1119-1122.

16 Alzheimer's Association. *"Early-Onset Dementia: A National Challenge, A Future Crisis."* Chicago, IL; 2006.

17 P. Kemper, H.L. Komisar, L. Alecxih, "Long-Term Care Over an Uncertain Future: What Can Current Retirees Expect?" *Inquiry* 42;2005:335–350.

18 E. O'Brien, "Medicaid and Long-Term Care." *Long-Term Care Financing Project: Fact Sheet,* Georgetown University (February 2007).

19 Kaiser Family Foundation, *Medicaid and Long-Term Care Services and Supports,* February 2009. Available at www.kff.org.

20 J.A. Cutler, B. Spillman, E.J. Tell, "Private Financing of Long-term Care: Market Penetration and Market Potential," *Academy Health Annual Research Meeting.* Boston, June 2010.

21 S.H. Kaye, C. Harrington, M.P. LaPlante, "Long-Term Care: Who Gets It, Who Provides It, Who Pays, And How Much?" *Health Affairs* 29(1);2010: 11-21.

22 College Board, *Trends in College Pricing 2009,* Washington, D.C., 2009.

23 C. Wolfson, D.B. Wolfson, M. Asgharian, et al, "A Reevaluation of the Duration of Survival After the Onset of Dementia," *The New England Journal of Medicine* 344(15); 2001: 1111-1115.

24 Institute of Medicine, *Retooling for an Aging America: Building the Health Care Workforce,* Washington D.C.: The National Academy of Sciences, 2008.

25 G. Kolata, "Promise Seen for Detection of Alzheimer's," The New York Times. June 23, 2010.

26 Alzheimer's Disease Education & Referral Center, *Alzheimer's Disease Medications: Fact Sheet,* Bethesda, MD: National Institutes of Health, Publication No. 08-3431; 2010, http://www.nia.nih.gov/NR/rdonlyres/5178456B-4E16-4A71-A704-46637C6FE61B/14990/ADMedsEnglishFINAL71410.pdf, accessed August 26, 2010.

27 Alzheimer's Association, *FDA-Approved Treatments for Alzheimer's,* Chicago, IL, 2007.

28 D.S. Geldmacher, "Cost-effectiveness of drug therapies for Alzheimer's disease: A brief review," *Neuropsychiatric Disease and Treatment.* 4.3 (2008): 549-555.

29 C. Wolfson, R. Oremus, V. Shukla, et al, "Donepezil and Rivastigmine in the Treatment of Alzheimer's Disease: A Best-Evidence Synthesis of the Published Data on Their Efficacy and Cost-Effectiveness," Clinical Therapuetics 24(6); 2002: 862-886.

30 A. Clegg, J. Bryant, T. Nicholson, et al, "Clinical and Cost-Effectiveness of Donepezil, Rivastigmine, and Galantamine for Alzheimer's Disease: A Systematic Review," *International Journal of Technology Assessment in Health Care* 18(3);2002:497-507.

31 K.M. Murphy, R.H. Topel, *Measuring the Gains from Medical Research: An Economic Approach.* The University of Chicago Press. Chicago, 2003.

32 E.R. Dorsey, J. de Roulet, J.P. Thompson, et al, "Funding of US Biomedical Research, 2003-2008," *Journal of the American Medical Association,* 303(2); 2010: 137-143.

33 National Institutes of Health, *Estimates of Funding for Various Research, Condition, and Disease Categories (RCDC),* http://report.nih.gov/rcdc/categories/#bpopup, February 2010. Accessed August 1, 2010.

34 National Institutes of Health Working Group on Priority Setting, *Setting Research Priorities at the National Institutes of Health,* Bethesda, MD: National Institutes of Health, 2001.

35 Alzheimer's Association, *Federal Priorities 2010,* Chicago, IL, 2010b.

36 Kaiser Family Foundation, *Health Care Reform and the CLASS Act,* April 2010. Available at www.kff.org.

37 National Health Policy Forum, *The Basics: The Community Living Assistance Services and Supports (CLASS) Act: Major Legislative Provisions,* The George Washington University. June 9, 2010.

38 Genworth Financial, *Cost of Care Survey: Home Care Providers, Adult Day Health Care Facilities, Assisted Living Facilities and Nursing Homes,* 2010.

39 L.R. Feinberg, S.L. Newman, L. Gray, K.N. Kolb, *The State of the States in Family Caregiver Support: A 50-State Study,* Washington, D.C.: Family Caregiver Alliance: National Center on Caregiving, 2004.

40 L. Simon-Rusinowitz, G.M. Garcia, D. Martin, et al, "Hiring Relatives as Caregivers in Two States: Developing an Education and Research Agenda for Policy Makers," *Social Work in Public Health.* 25; 2010: 17-41.

41 N. Johnson, P. Oliff, E. Williams, *An Update on State Budget Cuts,* Washington, D.C.: Center on Budget and Policy Priorities, 2010.

42 S.H. Kaye, M.P. LaPlante, C. Harrington, "Do Noninstitutional Long-Term Care Services Reduce Medicaid Spending?" *Health Affairs* 28(1);2009: 262-272.

43 J. Bynum, Characteristics, *Costs & Health Service Use For Medicare Beneficiaries with a Dementia Diagnosis,* The Dartmouth Institute for Health Policy and Clinical Care, March 22, 2009.

44 K.M. Langa, M.E. Chernew, M.U. Kabeto, et al, "National Estimates of the Quantity and Cost of Informal Caregiving for the Elderly with Dementia," *Journal of General Internal Medicine* 16; 2001: 770-778.

45 D.P. Rice, P.J. Fox, W. Max W, et al., "The Economic Burden of Alzheimer's Disease Care," *Health Affairs,* Summer;1993: 165-176.

a The increased annual health care costs per caregiver are estimated to be $530. This $530 per-caregiver cost was converted to an $800 per-Alzheimer's-patient cost. This conversion was based on there being 1.5 caregivers per person with Alzheimer's. The number of caregivers for individuals with dementia is estimated to be 11.2 million (Alzheimer's Association 2010a, updated to 2010). Approximately 70 percent of dementia cases are caused by Alzheimer's, resulting in 7.8 million caregivers for the 5.3 million individuals with Alzheimer's disease (Alzheimer's Association, 2010a).

b The annual net cost per Alzheimer's patient was not projected for 2050, because of the uncertainty of what medical technology will be available then.

c The financing of the formal care costs is based on Bynum's (2009) study of individuals with and without dementia, because that study showed the shares of costs by payer. The share of costs represented by informal care is based on the $27,200 average informal care estimate shown in Table 2. The share of costs represented by caregivers' increased health care costs is based on health care expenditure data by payer from the Centers for Medicare and Medicaid Services.

d Some of these informal care costs are borne by businesses, because caregivers who are employees have increased absenteeism and reduced productivity. In 2002, these costs were estimated to be $37 billion per year (Koppel R, Alzheimer's Disease: The Costs to U.S. Businesses in 2002, Alzheimer's Association. Department of Sociology, University of Pennsylvania. Philadelphia, PA 2002).

e These studies typically estimated the net costs for patients with dementia, which were assumed to be representative of the net costs for people with Alzheimer's disease.

f The studies estimating the net cost for informal care do not typically include control groups (McDaid D, "Estimating the costs of informal care for people with Alzheimer's disease: methodological and practical challenges." International Journal of Geriatric Psychiatry 16; 2001: 400-405), so informal care costs per individual may be over-estimated because elderly individuals without Alzheimer's disease require informal care as well.

ACKNOWLEDGMENTS

I am grateful to Charlene Harrington, RN, Ph.D., FAAN (professor emeritus of sociology and nursing, and director, UCSF National Center for Personal Assistance Services at the University of California, San Francisco); Richard M. Scheffler, Ph.D. (distinguished professor of health economics and public policy, School of Public Health and Richard & Rhoda Goldman School of Public Policy, University of California, Berkeley); and Mistique C. Felton, MPH (senior research associate, the Nicholas C. Petris Center on Health Care Markets and Consumer Welfare, School of Public Health, University of California, Berkeley) for their comments on an earlier draft of this chapter. I thank the McCormacks for their willingness to share their story about the impact of Alzheimer's disease on their family.

Are We Prepared?

What's the Workplace Impact?

Alzheimer's, Women and the American Work Force

- Working women get even less support for elder care than they do for child care. By large margins, they find it easier to find good child care than elder care. And 46 percent of working women say they've wanted time off from the job for Alzheimer care and couldn't get it.

- Workers providing Alzheimer care most crave flexibility in their work hours and schedules, as well as better or more Alzheimer care options for their loved ones living with the disease.

- Forty percent of caregivers care for a relative who would fall outside the allowable family members for whom a caregiver can take leaver under the Family and Medical Leave Act (FMLA).

- A significant majority of working caregivers of people with Alzheimer's—64 percent—reported the need to come in late, leave early or take time off as a result of their caregiving responsibilities. Another 20 percent reported that they needed to take a leave of absence to care for their family member with Alzheimer's disease.

- Workers providing care to a family member with Alzheimer's disease or other dementias were 31 percent more likely than other caregivers to reduce hours or quit if their family member had the disease but was not experiencing behavioral symptoms, and 68 percent more likely than other caregivers to reduce hours or quit if their family member was also experiencing behavioral symptoms.

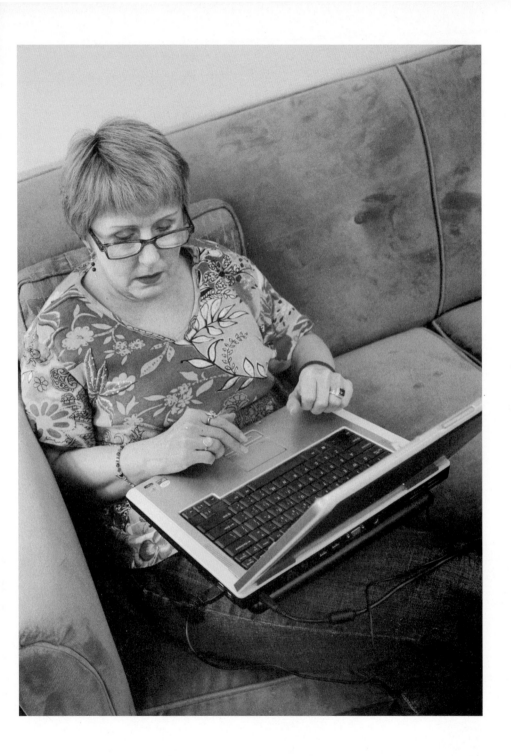

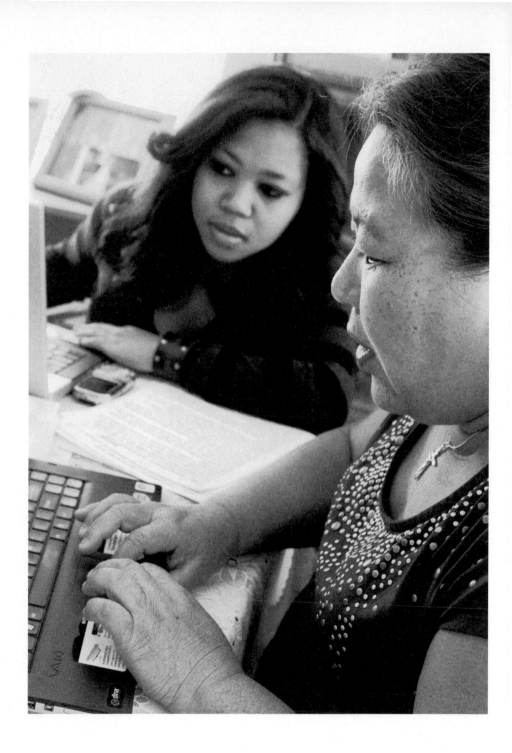

What's the Workplace Impact?

By Ann O'Leary

J ustice Sandra Day O'Connor, who retired from the Supreme Court in 2006, publicly reflected that she had wanted to stay on the court longer but needed to leave her job to provide care and comfort to her husband who was dying of Alzheimer's disease.[1] Former President Ronald Reagan retreated from public life and his ongoing work in 1994 when the progression of Alzheimer's disease made it impossible to continue his efforts.[2]

While these are the most high-profile cases of the impact of Alzheimer's disease on workers—both those caring for family members with Alzheimer's and those suffering from the disease themselves—such stories play out every day in the lives of many Americans. This chapter will:

- Explore how millions of workers are caught between the dual demands of work and providing care for a relative with Alzheimer's disease.

- Explain how too few workers have access to workplace policies and practices that support Alzheimer's caregivers, and how workplace policies for those living with the disease are nonexistent or underdeveloped.

- Show the trend of the rising number of workers being diagnosed with Alzheimer's disease while still in the workplace.

- Recommend solutions for addressing the impact of Alzheimer's in the workplace.

Alzheimer caregivers in the workplace

Alzheimer's disease will have an increasing impact on our workers and workplaces due to the dramatic demographic shift our population and our work force is experiencing. This demographic shift will require more workers to provide care for their family members who are living longer.

The U.S. Census Bureau predicts that the 65-and-older population will more than double from nearly 35 million in 2000 to over 71 million in 2030, going from 12 percent to nearly 20 percent of the population.[3] With more Americans living longer and the aging of the baby boomers, the incidence of Alzheimer's and other dementias is expected to increase because it is a disease that primarily impacts adults 65 years of age and older. By 2050, researchers predict that as many as 16 million individuals age 65 and older will be living with Alzheimer's disease, triple the number living with the disease today.[4]

Caregiving falls largely to those who must combine work in the paid labor force with being unpaid caregivers of family members.

This increase in the number of older Americans living with Alzheimer's—combined with a movement to deinstitutionalize elder care and a decrease in the government's commitment to pay for in-home care services for the elderly and disabled—means that more family members will be called upon to provide unpaid care and assistance to loved ones with Alzheimer's.[5]

As the demand for unpaid family care increases for individuals with Alzheimer's, fewer family caregivers will be available to provide the care. While, as mentioned, the population of Americans 65 and older is expected to nearly double by 2030, the population of typical caregivers—adult children ages 45 to 65—is expected to only increase by 25 percent in this same time period.[6]

The math just doesn't add up in terms of the ratio of caregivers to older Americans. In addition, most caregivers today must combine care with work, which makes caregiving all that more stressful. Today, women are half of all workers, and two-thirds of families are made up of dual-worker couples or single working heads of households.[7] This means caregiving falls largely to those who must combine work in the paid labor force with being unpaid caregivers of family members.

So while many women are no longer at home full-time, the vast majority of caregivers are still women. Sixty percent of all Alzheimer caregivers are women—6.7 million women. Of these women, 56 percent are working.[8] A 2010 study from the Families and Work Institute on working elder caregivers finds that all working caregivers of elderly family members are equally divided between men and women.[9] However, this does not appear to hold true for care providers of family members with Alzheimer's disease—a 2009 survey established that of the working Alzheimer care providers, 62 percent were women.[10]

What's more, today's generation of Alzheimer caregivers face unique challenges. With many women giving birth later in life, 37 percent of today's female caregivers are caring for both a family member with Alzheimer's disease and children under 18 years of age still living at home.[11] Many families also now live farther apart, and as a result, the Alzheimer's Association estimates that somewhere between just under 1 million to just over 1.5 million caregivers are providing "long-distance caregiving."[12]

The impact on work for Alzheimer caregivers

My professional life all but stopped. Finding doctors for him and getting him to appointments and coordinating escalating medical needs swallowed entire days.[13]

While the above sentiment was written by Jonathan Rauch, a journalist who was caring for his father who suffered from Parkinson's disease, it very well could have been written by my own mother. My mother quit her job last year—just six months shy of turning 66, the age to qualify for full Social Security benefits—because she could no longer manage the care needs of her mother who was suffering from dementia yet trying to stay in her own home. A doctor's appointment rescheduled at the last moment. A fall. A paid-care provider who called in sick. An angry incident between my confused grandmother and the care provider. Each of these episodes sent my mother into further career crisis. Unable to manage her work and satisfy the needs of her employer, she finally just felt she had to call it quits and retire early.

My mother is not alone. The impact of providing care to a family member with Alzheimer's disease or other dementias causes severe strain on one's ability to work effectively. According to the working elder caregiver study from the Families and Work Institute, a majority of working caregivers of the elderly (54 percent) report interference between caregiving and work, and one in five current caregivers report experiencing a negative impact at work as a result of this interference.[14] The Alzheimer's Association's new Women and Alzheimer's poll found that a significant majority of working caregivers of people with Alzheimer's—61 percent—reported the need to come in late, leave early or take time off as a result of their caregiving responsibilities.[15] Another 20 percent reported that they needed to take a leave of absence to care for their family member with Alzheimer's disease.[16]

More than 60 percent of working caregivers of people with Alzheimer's reported the need to come in late, leave early or take time off as a result of their caregiving responsibilities.

Some, like my mother, found it impossible to stay in the labor force at the same level. The Alzheimer's Association Women and Alzheimer's poll found that more than a third (34 percent) of women caregivers of people with Alzheimer's had to give up their job.[17] This number is much larger than overall estimates for elder caregivers. According to the 1999 MetLife Juggling Act study, 16 percent of working caregivers quit their jobs.[18] A 2009 survey conducted by the National Alliance for Caregiving and the AARP found that among all caregivers, 10 percent had to quit work or take early retirement.[19] The larger percentage of Alzheimer caregivers quitting their jobs is consistent with other research contrasting Alzheimer caregivers with other elder caregivers. Another study found that caregivers providing care to a family member with Alzheimer's disease or other dementias were 31 percent more likely than other caregivers to reduce hours or quit if their family member had the disease but was not experiencing behavioral symptoms, and 68 percent more likely to reduce hours or quit than other caregivers if their family member was also experiencing behavioral symptoms.[20]

Workplace policies for working caregivers

These numbers make one thing very clear: Working caregivers of family members with Alzheimer's disease need time and resources to deal with the challenges of providing care and working. The overwhelming majority—61 percent—need flexibility in their work schedules and time off to provide care. While we don't know the exact reasons that over one-third of working women who are Alzheimer caregivers are quitting their jobs, we do know that certain workplace policies help caregivers stay employed while taking the time needed to care for their loved ones.

With nearly half of all workers expecting to be providing family care for an elder in the next five years, according to the working elder caregiving study by the Families and Work

FIGURE 1 : The effect of caregiving on work:

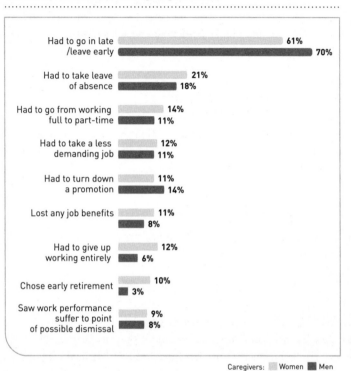

Caregivers: Women Men

Institute, these policies are important for all elder caregivers. But the difference between Alzheimer caregivers and other elder caregivers is that the disease often requires
the provision of family care for many years. Forty-three percent of caregivers of people
with Alzheimer's disease have been providing care for one to four years compared to 33
percent of other elder caregivers.[21] In addition, Alzheimer's is an unpredictable disease,
particularly at the early stages. The longevity and unpredictability put a greater burden
on working caregivers for the time and financial resources necessary to fully support
their family members.

This section will explore the state of existing policies to support workers with Alzheimer
caregiving responsibilities by examining federal laws and government programs. It then
will highlight voluntary employer practices, including best practices offered by employers
to aid workers in balancing work with caring for a family member with Alzheimer's.

Government policies to aid working caregivers

According to the newest Alzheimer's Association poll, workers caring for elder family members most crave flexibility in their work hour and schedules, as well as better or more Alzheimer care options for their loved ones living with the disease.[22]

Flexibility for working caregivers

Flexibility is the number-one wish of elder caregivers—flexibility to set hours, reduce their schedules or change the location of their workplace—or combine flexibility alternatives to make work fit with their needs while providing care to their family member with Alzheimer's disease.[23]

> *Workers caring for elder family members most crave flexibility in their work hours and schedules, as well as better or more Alzheimer care options for their loved ones living with the disease.*

We know from the Families and Work Institute's National Study of Employers that most employees have scant access to workplace flexibility—particularly the flexibility needed by caregivers of family members with Alzheimer's. Most Alzheimer caregivers report the need to come in late or leave early. Yet only 37 percent of employers report that they periodically allow most or all employees to change start and quitting times, and only 10 percent allow most or all employees to change starting or quitting times on a daily basis.[24] Other caregivers report the need to reduce hours, yet only 13 percent of employers allow most or all of their employees to move from full-time to part-time and back again while remaining in the same position or level.[25]

To date, there is no law requiring employers to offer flexible or predictable work schedules, and these numbers show that not very many businesses voluntarily offer flexibility. In the previous *Shriver Report* and a follow-up report titled *Our Working Nation*, Heather Boushey and I recommended that Congress require employers to set up a process to allow employees the right to request flexible or predictable schedules. This would spark conversations about the needs of employers and employees and protect workers with the right to ask for flexibility.[26] The ability to set up a system of flexibility is particularly important for caregivers of people with Alzheimer's, who may need to set up flexible schedules—and possibly revise them—over many years as they balance work and long-term care.

Time off to provide family care

Family and Medical Leave Act

The Family and Medical Leave Act (FMLA) is a powerful tool for family members caring for loved ones with Alzheimer's. It allows for covered workers to take up to 12 weeks of unpaid leave per year, which can be taken through reduced schedules or intermittent leave, to care for a spouse or parent with Alzheimer's disease.[27] This provides important flexibility to allow workers to take job-protected leave in order to provide the continual, long-term family care that Alzheimer's disease often demands. Twelve weeks of leave taken intermittently or as a reduced schedule allows workers to be creative. For example, a worker could take FMLA leave for one day a week for the entire year or for 1.5 hours per day for the entire year to provide care to a family member with Alzheimer's. Or, as another example, a family member providing long-distance care could take three days off at 20 different times in the year to provide care to a spouse or parent with Alzheimer's disease.

Forty percent of Alzheimer caregivers are providing care to a relative not covered under the Family and Medical Leave Act.

However, the law falls short in several key respects for working caregivers of family member's with Alzheimer's.[28] First, the definition of family is limited to care for children, parents and spouses. This means that a worker cannot take leave to care for a parent-in-law, a grandparent or another relative with Alzheimer's disease. Yet according to the newest Alzheimer's Association poll, 40 percent of caregivers are providing care to a relative who would fall outside the allowable family members for whom a caregiver can take leaver under the FMLA, including grandparents, siblings, in-laws, aunts and uncles.[29] The FMLA also only covers about half of all U.S. workers due to eligibility requirements for workers and size requirements for employers.[30] Because FMLA does not cover these caregivers, they are at the mercy of their employer when they need to take leave for work to provide care.

Second, the law allows employers to require their workers to substitute any of their accrued paid vacation leave, personal leave or family leave for FMLA leave. This means that some worn-out working caregivers only get leave to care for their family member with Alzheimer's disease and have no time left over for a vacation day to restore their own energy and health, or a sick day to recover from their own illness. This limitation is particularly troubling given the finding from the newest Alzheimer's Association poll showing that 68 percent of women Alzheimer caregivers report emotional stress, and 51 percent report physical stress from caregiving.[31]

Finally, the FMLA is unpaid, a financial burden that is particularly challenging for caregivers who must miss work or reduce their hours, sometimes for years, as they care for their ailing relative with Alzheimer's.

Income and retirement savings replacement

The newest Alzheimer's Association poll also showed that the majority of working Alzheimer caregivers, 55 percent, were the primary breadwinners of the household, which means that quitting or reducing hours with no wage replacement would cause a severe strain on the family.[32]

Paid family leave

Two states—California and New Jersey—have programs that provide wage replacement for workers taking leave to care for a family member with Alzheimer's disease. Both programs allow six weeks of wage replacement if your employer provides leave, and allow it to be taken on an intermittent basis.[33] President Obama proposed a 2011 budget that includes funding to allow new states to develop paid family leave programs and to expand the reach of the programs in existing states.

The majority of working Alzheimer caregivers are the primary breadwinners of their household.

The need for income replacement while Alzheimer caregivers are temporarily out of work caring for their ill family members is crucial, as demonstrated by Brent Fulton's chapter on the economic impact of Alzheimer's disease. These programs are an important first step, but they could be strengthened. For starters, California and New Jersey should boost efforts to spread the word to workers about these programs. Currently, awareness is very low that these programs are available and can be used for caregiving. For example, in a 2007 survey, only 28 percent of Californians knew about the California paid family leave program.[34]

Furthermore, these paid-leave programs offering wage replacement should be coupled with FMLA protection—requiring employers to allow workers to take leave and to provide them the same job upon their return. Right now, state paid-leave programs allow many more workers to qualify for the leave than to qualify for FMLA. That means many workers are unable to access the paid-leave program because their employers won't give them the time off to provide the care in the first place.

Social Security credit

In addition to lost wages, working caregivers—particularly women who may have taken time away from the workplace to care for children—lose the ability to earn credits to qualify for Social Security when they take time off to provide care for a relative with Alzheimer's disease. While Social Security provides some protection for married women by allowing women to receive 50 percent of their husband's Social Security benefits, it leaves too few women with little resources in retirement. Representative Nita Lowey (D-N.Y.) has introduced a bill that would allow workers to earn Social Security credits for up to five years when providing unpaid care for an average of 80 hours a month.[35] This proposal would help workers—who are disproportionately women—take leave to provide care while not sacrificing their own retirement security to do so.

Financial support to provide paid caregivers

In-home health and support services

While time off to provide direct family care is essential, it is often not enough. Family members with Alzheimer's disease often need round-the-clock attention. To ensure fewer work disruptions, working caregivers need support for paid home healthcare services. In fact, the newest Alzheimer's Association poll found that workers most wanted more or better care options for their loved ones.[36] Care options, outside family caregivers, can provide great relief to family members and allow caregivers to stay in the work force. In one study of government expenditures for formal residential and home-help for the elderly, researchers found that an increase in paid elder caregiving increased the labor force participation rates of women by relieving their informal care burden.[37] Unfortunately, state budget cuts threaten paid caregiving services by withdrawing state Medicaid funds for such services.[38]

Dependent care tax credit

In addition to the financial burden of missing work to provide care, many working caregivers of Alzheimer's disease spend their own resources to provide care while they are at work. Unlike funding paid for child care, Alzheimer and elder caregivers receive no tax relief for the funds that they spend in this way. Heather Boushey and I previously recommended that Congress consider expanding the Child and Dependent Tax Credit, or create an independent caregiving credit, to allow workers to receive some tax relief for caregiving expenses even when the person in need of care doesn't live with the caregiver and is not entirely financially dependent.[39]

Business policies to aid working caregivers

Businesses do not need to wait for government action to provide their workers with the policies discussed above. In fact, many do so on their own. The most common workplace policies offered by employers to accommodate employee elder caregiving needs include time off to provide care without losing one's job (75 percent of employers), eldercare resource and referral services (31 percent) and dependent care savings accounts (23 percent).[40]

As discussed earlier, the provision of time off and flexibility is very uneven for workers. Too few have the protection afforded by our existing laws, and too few businesses offer these benefits on their own accord. The essay by Cathleen Benko and Anne Weisberg in this book offers one promising model of how to provide needed flexibility for workers across their careers, a model built on rewarding employees on their career results.

One of the most promising resource and referral workplace practices to support working caregivers caring for a family member with Alzheimer's is an employer-provided geriatric care manager. Research has shown that employers that provide intensive geriatric care manager services—individualized services to employees to help with care planning from arranging adult daycare or assisted living services to answering questions about the progression of the disease to helping explain insurance coverage—had positive outcomes for their employees and their business.[41] Their employees were more on-task and healthier over time.[42] For example:

- IBM offers its employees six hours per year of paid elder services such as care management in the form of a geriatric nurse or social worker who conducts home assessments, develops a home care plan and researches the availability, costs and quality of alternative housing.

- Time, Inc., provides a medical-decision support program that gets employees in touch with a medical researcher and a physician who share the latest research about diseases such as Alzheimer's.[43]

Much more can be done by the government and private employers to provide the needed supports—from time off to informational and financial resources—to aid caregivers of family members with Alzheimer's disease. The long-term and unpredictable nature of Alzheimer caregiving takes dedicated and ongoing negotiations between employers and employees to ensure that the needs of both parties are met. A way to ensure that these conversations take place would be to require businesses to allow employees the job-protected right to request flexibility.

Workers with Alzheimer's disease

The challenges associated with the millions of working caregivers who are balancing work and care have had the largest impact on workplaces to date. But workers with Alzheimer's disease will become an increasing presence in the work force in the years ahead, creating new challenges that workplaces are not yet prepared to handle.

Two sets of workers face Alzheimer's disease while still working. First, workers who have younger-onset Alzheimer's disease—Alzheimer's diagnosed before the age of 65—are most likely to still be in the work force because workers under 65 years of age have a higher work force participation rate in the general population than older workers. Up to 130,000 individuals with younger-onset Alzheimer's disease could face this diagnosis while still working.[44]

Second, individuals over the age of 65 who have Alzheimer's disease could still be working when they receive their diagnosis. Currently, the number of individuals over 65 who have Alzheimer's disease while still working could be as high as 464,000 but could increase to as high as 848,000 by 2050 because older workers are staying in the work force longer.[45]

Aiding workers with Alzheimer's disease

Alzheimer's disease ultimately forces individuals to withdraw from the work force. But the path to leaving the work force can be a difficult one—both for workers and for employers. This section will outline the challenges that workers and employers face as a result of ill-fitting laws and social policies, and a lack of model practices to aid employers.

Workers may begin experiencing symptoms of Alzheimer's disease—short-term memory loss, language problems and loss of knowledge, difficulties in planning and organization, impaired decision making and accompanying anxiety and depression[46]—long before knowing what is wrong or receiving a diagnosis. This problem is especially true for individuals with younger-onset Alzheimer's disease, as colleagues, family members and even medical professionals often don't expect Alzheimer's in a person who is in his or her 40s or 50s; thus, a diagnosis can take months or even years.[47] Employers may be faced with a worker who was once a reliable and strong member of the work force becoming increasingly unable to perform, and the employer may not have the tools to discuss the problem with the worker in a constructive way. In many instances, neither the employer nor the worker knows the nature of the problem, but they do recognize that the worker can no longer perform and, as a result, in two-thirds of the cases the employer fires the worker or the worker voluntarily quits, often causing great financial hardship to the worker and his or her family.[48]

Americans with Disabilities Act

Alzheimer's disease does not fit neatly into our main law protecting people with disabilities for workplace discrimination, the Americans with Disabilities Act (ADA). Title I of the ADA prohibits employers from discriminating against qualified applicants or employees with disabilities and requires employers to provide necessary reasonable accommodations to enable qualified workers with disabilities to participate in and enjoy equal employment opportunities. However, a number of barriers exist for workers with Alzheimer's disease to access their rights under the ADA.

First, workers must recognize that they have a disability, defined as substantial limitation in performing a major life activity, in order to request and receive accommodations. When symptoms arise, it may take time before the worker recognizes that there is a problem and, even then, as noted earlier, the road to diagnosis is often a long one. In fact, according to a study conducted for the U.S. Preventative Services Task Force, two-thirds of primary care physicians misdiagnose the disease in their younger patients.[49]

While an exact diagnosis of Alzheimer's disease is not necessary to receive an accommodation, the employee must nonetheless establish that she has a medical condition that is limiting her ability to perform a major life activity and that it cannot be corrected with a mitigating measure.[50] Requesting and receiving an accommodation for symptoms arising from Alzheimer's disease without a correct diagnosis could be challenging. For example, if an employee is misdiagnosed with depression and given medication to mitigate the depression, the employee may try to continue working and ask for no accommodation with the hopes that the medication would correct the problem.

The delay in asking for accommodation and continuing frustration by the worker who is not getting better could ultimately lead to a termination of employment. As one worker aptly stated, "By the time I was given a diagnosis, I had had several years of failing at my job, been forced to retire, become penniless. Had I had a diagnosis, (my employer) would have been legally bound to give me a lesser job. What a waste!"[51]

Second, if and when a worker receives the diagnosis, he or she must still be qualified for the job and able to conduct it with reasonable accommodations. At least one court has noted that there are no reasonable accommodations for Alzheimer's disease: "If the plaintiff did, indeed, have Alzheimer's disease, the defendants would not be liable pursuant to the ADA for their decision to terminate his employment because no reasonable accommodation would have been possible."[52] This may be true for many workers with Alzheimer's disease because by the time they receive the diagnosis, their cognitive impairment is so great that they may be unable to perform their job even with accommodations.[53]

The Equal Employment Opportunity Commission (EEOC) puts out guidance for employers and employees to ensure that workers who have specific diseases—including epilepsy, diabetes, cancer and intellectual disabilities (previously known as mental retardation)—are not discriminated against and receive appropriate accommodations.[54] No such guidance exists to aid employers of workers who have degenerative cognitive disabilities, such as Alzheimer's and other dementias. Such guidance could be particularly helpful for employers who suspect that their employee has Alzheimer's disease but do not know how to approach their employee to offer support and guidance. The EEOC should consider putting out guidance that helps employers and employees with each stage of Alzheimer's disease in the workplace—the detection of the problem; the diagnosis of the disability; the accommodation, where still possible, of workers who would like, and are able, to remain in the work force; and the aid for employees who ultimately must transition out of the work force when they can no longer perform their job even with reasonable accommodations.

Given the potential for a rising numbers of workers who may receive such diagnosis while in the work force, this guidance would have a tremendous impact on employers and employees dealing with Alzheimer's—both in providing accommodations while the individual is still able to work and in aiding employers in how to help employees to effectively transition out of the workplace. In addition, guidance on accommodations could aid those workers in staying on the job for a little longer, which benefits both the employer and the employee. For the employer, it can allow the worker to pass on their institutional knowledge before losing their memory and can ensure that a replacement worker is well trained.[55] For the employee, it can mean additional income and more time in which the person remains engaged in the work that may have defined her before the disease struck.

Social Security Disability Insurance

For all workers with Alzheimer's disease, they will ultimately need to stop working, and when they do, they will need financial support to replace their income from their job in order to sustain themselves and their family.

Workers who are permanently disabled qualify for Social Security Disability Insurance (SSDI). In March 2010, the Social Security Administration (SSA) expanded its list of Compassionate Allowances, which allow individuals with certain diseases and medical conditions to quickly qualify for disability insurance, to include early-onset Alzheimer's disease (also known as younger-onset Alzheimer's disease, with both terms referring to those individuals diagnosed under the age of 65).[56] This change will mean that workers with early-onset Alzheimer's disease who previously may have had to wait years to qualify for SSDI—awaiting the progression of the disease yet unable to work—will be able to qualify within a matter of months.

Employers and workers need more information both about workplace accommodations for individuals with Alzheimer's disease who are still able to remain in the workplace and about the availability of SSDI for workers no longer able to work due to early-onset Alzheimer's disease. The EEOC and the SSA should team up to provide joint guidance to employers and workers on both ADA workplace accommodations, as well as the availability of qualifying for SSDI through the Compassionate Allowances program.

Model employer practices

With little guidance from the government on what to do when faced with an employee who has increasing cognitive decline, employers are left on their own to determine how to support their employees. Often, with no experience in doing so, they simply fire the employee as the employee becomes progressively unable to work. But there are steps that can be taken. First and foremost, employers should be encouraged to urge their employees to seek medical attention when they notice cognitive decline in the workplace. Once a diagnosis is made, the employer should actively work with employees in either creating an accommodation plan or accessing both private disability insurance available through the employer and, once they leave the workforce, SSDI.

Conclusion

Alzheimer's disease already impacts workplaces across the country due to the millions of workers who are combining work with unpaid care of a family member or friend with Alzheimer's disease. Our laws and the voluntary practices of businesses have room to be improved—to expand the reach of paid leave, job-protected leave, workplace flexibility and resources for caregivers—in order to help caregivers remain financially stable and effectively able to work and provide care. Alzheimer's disease may also soon have a larger impact on workplaces that employ workers living with the disease. The challenges of providing appropriate accommodation and transition plans are real, and the government should do more to ensure that employers and employees understand the rights of employees diagnosed with Alzheimer's disease.

ENDNOTES

1   James M. Klatell, "O'Connor Wanted to Stay on Bench Longer," CBS News, February 4, 2007, available at: http://www.cbsnews.com/stories/2007/02/04/national/main2430379.shtml?tag=contentMain;conten tBody (last accessed September 2010).

2   Lou Cannon, "Actor, Governor, President, Icon," *The Washington Post,* June 6, 2004, p. A28.

3   U.S. Census Bureau, "State Interim Population Projects by Age and Sex, Table B1, Interim Projections of the Population by Selected Age Groups for the United States and States: April 1, 2000 to July 1, 2030," available at http://www.census.gov/population/www/projections/files/SummaryTabB1.pdf (last accessed September 2010)

4   L.E. Hebert and others, "Alzheimer's Disease in the U.S. Population: Prevalence Estimates Using the 2000 Census," *Archives of Neurology* 60(2003):1119-1122, p. 1121.

5   Beverly B. Koerin, Marcia P. Harrigan and Mary Secret, "Eldercare and Employed Caregivers: A Public/ Private Responsibility?" *Journal of Gerontological Social Work,* 51 (1/2) (2008): 143-161.

6   Katherine Mack and Lee Thompson with Robert Friedland, "Data Profiles, Family Caregivers of Older Persons: Adult Children" (Washington: The Center on an Aging Society, Georgetown University, 2005).

7   Heather Boushey and Ann O'Leary, eds., *The Shriver Report: A Woman's Nation Changes Everything* (Washington: Center for American Progress, 2009).

8   Unpublished data from the 2009 National Alliance for Caregiving (NAC)/AARP survey of caregiving in the U.S., prepared under contract for the Alzheimer's Association by Matthew Greenwald and Associates, April 8, 2010 (hereinafter Alzheimer's Association, "Caregiving in the U.S. 2009.").

9   Kerstin Aumann and others, "Working Family Caregivers of the Elderly: Everyday Realities and Wishes for Change" (New York: Families and Work Institute, 2010).

10   Calculations based on Alzheimer's Association, "Caregiving in the U.S. 2009." This data showed that even though the percentage of male caregivers working is higher than female caregivers workers (67 percent compared to 56 percent), the percentage of working caregivers still skews toward more women because there are many more female caregivers (66 percent of caregivers are women). There are approximately 4.1 million female working caregivers compared to 2.6 million male working caregivers, which means that 62 percent of working caregivers are women.

11 Ibid.

12 Alzheimer's Association, *2010 Alzheimer's Disease Facts and Figures* (2010).

13 Jonathan Rauch, "Letting Go of My Father." *The Atlantic,* April, 2010.

14 Aumann and others, "Working Family Caregivers of the Elderly."

15 Alzheimer's Association, "Women & Alzheimer's Poll" (2010)..

16 Ibid.

17 Ibid.

18 MetLife Mature Market Institute, "The MetLife Juggling Act Study: Balancing Caregiving with Work and the Costs Involved" (1999).

19 Alzheimer's Association, "Caregiving in the U.S. 2009."

20 Alzheimer's Association, *2010 Alzheimer's Disease Facts and Figures,* fn 75 (citing Covnisky, KI; Eng, C; Liu L-Y; Sands, LP; Sehgal, AR; Walter, LC; et al. "Reduced Employment in Caregivers of Frail Elders: Impact of Ethnicity, Patient Clinical Characteristics and Caregiver Characteristics," *Journal of Gerontology: Medical Sciences* 56A(11) (2001): M707-713).

21 Alzheimer's Association, *2010 Alzheimer's Disease Facts and Figures* (2010).

22 Alzheimer's Association, "Women & Alzheimer's Poll" (2010)..

23 Aumann and others, "Working Family Caregivers of the Elderly."

24 Ellen Galinsky and others, "2008: National Study of Employers" (New York: Families and Work Institute, 2008).

25 Ibid.

26 Heather Boushey and Ann O'Leary, eds., *The Shriver Report: A Woman's Nation Changes Everything;* Heather Boushey and Ann O'Leary, "Our Working Nation: How Working Women are Reshaping America's Families and Economy and What it Means for Policymakers" (Washington: Center for American Progress, 2010).

27 29 U.S.C. § 2612 (2006). FMLA regulations specify Alzheimer's disease as an example of a serious health condition requiring continuing treatment by a medical provider, which is an allowable reason for a spouse or parent to take leave in order to provide care. 29 C.F.R. 825.115(d)

28 See, generally, Peggie R. Smith, "Elder Care, Gender and Work: The Work-Family Issue of the 21st Century," *Berkeley Journal of Employment and Labor Law* 25 (2004): 351; Aumann and others, "Working Family Caregivers of the Elderly."

29 Alzheimer's Association, "Women & Alzheimer's Poll" (2010).

30 U.S. Department of Labor, "Balancing the Needs of Families and Employers: Family and Medical Leave Surveys" (2000).

31 Alzheimer's Association, "Women & Alzheimer's Poll" (2010).

32 Ibid.

33 California Unemployment Insurance Code § 3301; New Jersey Statutes, Pensions and Retirement and Unemployment Compensation, Title 43A:21-38 and 39.

34 Ruth Milkman, "New Data on Paid Family Leave" (Los Angeles: UCLA Institute for Research on Labor and Employment, 2008).

35 H.R. 769, Social Security Caregiver Credit Act of 2009.

36 Alzheimer's Association, "Women & Alzheimer's Poll" (2010).

37 Tarja K. Viitanen, "Informal and Formal Care in Europe" (Germany: Forschungsinstitut zur Zukunft der Arbeit Institute for Study of Labor, 2007).

38 In 2010, at least 29 States and the District of Columbia are cutting home care services for low-income and disabled residents. *See* Nicole Johnson and others, "An Update on State Budget Cuts: At least 46 States Have Imposed Cuts that Hurt Vulnerable Residents and the Economy," (Washington: Center for Budget and Policy Priorities, 2010).

39 Heather Boushey and Ann O'Leary, "Our Working Nation."

40 Ellen Galinsky and others, "2008: National Study of Employers."

41 Donna L. Wagner, "Workplace Programs for Family Caregivers: Good Business and Good Practice" (San Francisco: Family Caregiver Alliance, 2003).

42 LifeCare, Inc., "Corporate Eldercare Programs: Their Impact, Effectiveness and the Implications for Employers" (2008).

43 Leah Dobkin, "How to Confront Elder Care Challenge," *Workforce Management,* April 2007, available at http://www.workforce.com/section/hr-management/feature/how-confront-elder-care-challenge/index.html (last accessed September 2010).

44 Approximately 65 percent of all individuals age 55 to 64 are still in the workforce. If individuals with early-onset Alzheimer's disease, 200,000 total, were in the workforce at the same rate, 130,000 would be in the workforce when they received the diagnosis. However, this number would quickly drop upon on set of disabling cognitive impairments. Only 22 percent of workers with such impairments remain in the workforce, which would be approximately 28,600 individuals with early-onset Alzheimer's. Figures derived from Health and Retirement Survey of 2000 as reported in Alzheimer's Association, *Early Onset Dementia: A National Challenge, A Future Crisis* (2006).

45 Only 300,000 to 500,000 individuals between the ages of 65 and 74 have Alzheimer's disease and this number is not projected to increase by 2050. The number of individuals 75 to 84 with Alzheimer's disease is 2.4 million in 2010 and is expected to double to 4.8 million by 2050. See L.E. Hebert and others, "Alzheimer's Disease in the U.S. Population," p. 1121. In 2007, the work participation rate of individuals who were 65 and older was 16 percent. See Bureau of Labor Statistics, "Spotlight on Statistics, Older Workers, July 2008, Chart Data," available at http://www.bls.gov/spotlight/2008/older_workers/data.htm#chart_02 (last accessed September 2010). Work participation rates are not broken down further by older age categories. Work participation rates are continuing to climb for older Americans, but given that we don't have the breakdown of the participation rate of our oldest workers, I conservatively estimate a constant rate of 16 percent workforce participation for those in the 65 and older category and derive the high numbers by taking 16 percent of the numbers of individuals with Alzheimer's disease in the 65 to 84 categories.

46 Drawn from Daniel Marson, "The Impact of Alzheimer's Disease on the Capacity to Work," Compassionate Allowance Hearing on Early Onset Alzheimer's Disease and Related Dementias, Social Security Administration, July 29, 2009 (hereinafter Marson presentation).

47 Alzheimer's Association, *Early-Onset Dementia: A National Challenge, A Future Crisis* (2006).

48 Ibid.

49 Beth Baker, "When Alzheimer's Strikes," *Compensation, Benefits & Rewards,* November 2008.

50 Equal Opportunity Employment Commission, Facts About the Americans with Disabilities Act, available at: www.eeoc.gov/facts/fs-ada.html (last accessed September 2010).

51 Alzheimer's Association, *Early-Onset Dementia: A National Challenge,* A Future Crisis (2006).

52 *Fink v. Printed Circuit Corp.,* 204 F. Supp. 2d 119, 129-30 (D. Mass., 2002).

53 Marson presentation.

54 U.S. Equal Employment Opportunity Commission, "Disability Discrimination, The Questions and Answers Series," available at: http://www.eeoc.gov/laws/types/disability.cfm (last accessed September 2010).

55 Baker *supra* note 49.

56 Social Security Administration, Compassionate Allowances, available at: http://www.socialsecurity.gov/compassionateallowances/ (last accessed September 2010).

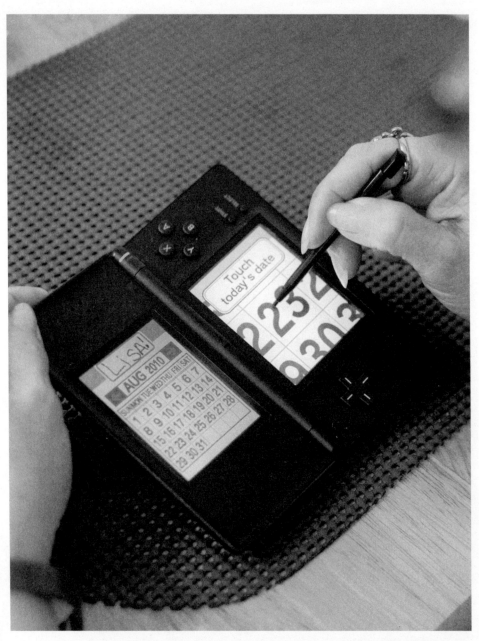

Lisa Carbo believes in keeping her mind stimulated with brain games on her Nintendo DS.

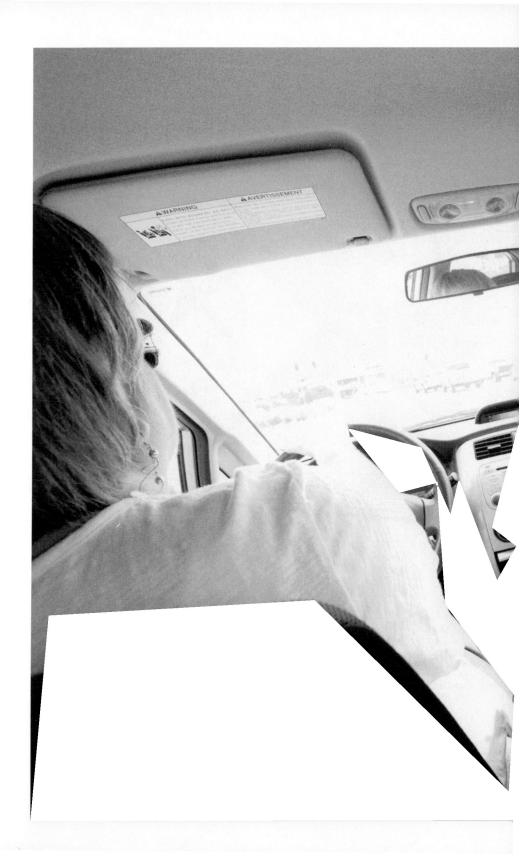

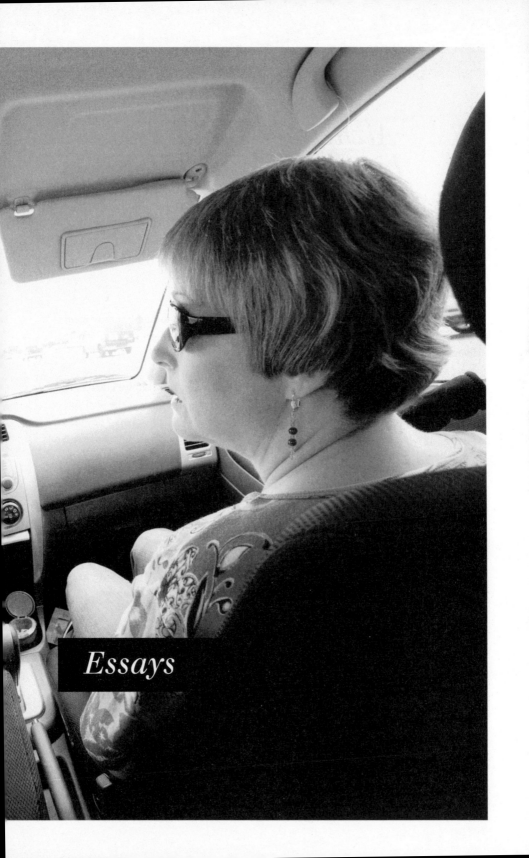

Essays

Alzheimer's and the Lattice Organization

By Cathleen Benko, vice chairman and chief talent officer, Deloitte LLP, and Anne Weisberg, director of talent, Deloitte Services LP, specializing in creating inclusive work environments

*W*e're a nation of working caregivers, and increasingly we're caring for family members with Alzheimer's. As a result, organizations today can no longer afford to ignore the eldercare issues of their employees.

"The role of the employer is huge in this whole conversation, now that we know that almost half of the work force has provided elder care at some point over the past five years, and this trend will only increase with the aging of the baby boomers," says Ellen Galinsky, president of the Families and Work Institute. "We are all going to have to learn how to handle aging in America."[1]

But what is the appropriate organizational response?

For the most part, companies have responded to the growing demand for elder care by expanding existing work/life benefits, originally designed to address child care, to include elder care. Over the decade between 1998 and 2008, the percentage of employers providing access to information about services for elderly family members grew from 23 to 39 percent.[2]

For example, Deloitte's* resource and referral program provides eldercare information, both by phone and online, to hundreds of Deloitte personnel every year. In line with this trend, several years ago Deloitte expanded its back-up care benefit—designed originally for personnel to use when their regular child day care fell through—to include elder care, and refers to the program now as back-up dependent day care. Another benefit offered by roughly two-thirds of best-in-class companies is several days off per year to care for an elderly relative without losing pay or having to use vacation days.[3]

However, while these work/life benefits are valuable and a step in the right direction, they do not address the multitude of challenges employees with eldercare issues face in fitting their work into their lives and their lives into their work as their needs change over time.

Patricia Romeo's story illustrates what happens when there is no systemic response. In 1990, she was leading recruiting for Deloitte Consulting LLP when she learned that she was pregnant with her first child and that her mother had Alzheimer's. As Patricia recounts, "Alzheimer's is such a challenging disease, and the demands on the caregiver are extremely unpredictable. There were fire drills all the time. I remember one such moment, several years after my daughter was born, when we were waiting for the elevator to take my mother to a doctor's appointment. I had my 3-year-old with me, and my mother had the mental capacity of a 3-year-old. She got on the wrong elevator, and we had to lock down the whole building because I had no way of knowing what she would do. Just when you think you have it under control, something would happen like that."

Despite a husband who had a flexible work situation and therefore shared child care, and siblings who lived in the same city and could help with their mother's care, Patricia felt she had no choice but to step out of the work force completely for five years to help care for her mother. As she says, "At the time, Deloitte was growing like crazy, and there were huge demands from the business that I knew I couldn't meet given the demands from caring for my mother."[4]

There were fewer options then. After her mother died, Patricia found a position at another company, but "I had to start over again from the bottom." Ultimately, 10 years after she left, Patricia came back to Deloitte and today leads their internal social networking site called D Street. But she can't help but wonder what her career would have been like if she hadn't had to step out and then step back in—and for over 10 years, Deloitte lost a valuable employee who knew the business and its people.

An organizational response to Patricia's story starts with recognizing that, far from an isolated incident, it is increasingly the norm. This fundamental shift is the result of a multitude of converging trends from significant changes in the family structure, to a critical mass of primary-breadwinner-women in the work force, and even the proliferation and advancement of technologies that provide new options—and challenges—for when, where and how work is done. In short, the work force is becoming more diverse along every dimension with increasing variation in what any one individual needs at any point in time, and even what that same individual may need over time. As a result, career and life can no longer be bucketed into separate realms.

When elder care is added to the lengthening list of changing work force needs, it is clear that a more comprehensive, systemic response is required. Kathleen Christiansen, director of the Program on Workplace, Workforce and Working Families at the Alfred P. Sloan Foundation, has funded research on work-life for over 20 years, and as she says, "Employers will need a new template to think about elder care, because it is not the same as child care. Given the variability and unpredictability of elder care, and the emotional as well as physical toll it takes, the eldercare template has to consider how to fit the needs of employees with how work gets done and the impact to their careers of taking time to perform elder care. There is no one single way to approach the eldercare needs of the work force."

Rather than a one-size-fits-all approach, therefore, organizations must employ what we call the Corporate Lattice™ model. In contrast with the rigid, linear corporate ladder model, which has been the prevailing model for how companies manage their work and their people, the lattice model provides a more adaptive, flexible view of how work gets done, how careers are built and how participation is fostered. At the heart of the lattice organization is a customized workplace that provides agility and options for both employees and employers. Lattice organizations create a variety of career paths for individuals—paths that move up, down, diagonally and across. This allows those people who choose to do so to dial down their career progression or plateau for a period to care for family members with Alzheimer's (among other needs), without completely falling out of the work force.

Similarly, lattice organizations take advantage of today's abundance of options for how, when and where work is done—through teleworking and work schedules that are customized rather than the standard 9 to 5 in the office. For employees dealing with Alzheimer's, lattice ways to work afford greater flexibility to continue to contribute at work while also caring for their loved ones. Lastly, lattice organizations encourage people to create communities of support around particular issues, such as caring for family members with Alzheimer's. That not only helps those in the community connect to each other but also creates a greater sense of connection between them and the organization.

For employers, these options create flexibility and drive greater employee engagement and loyalty, resulting in superior performance. The lattice organization understands that talent practices must be aligned with business operations to deliver both high performance and career-life fit.

Becki Horton's story exemplifies how Deloitte's journey to become a lattice organization has helped her manage an intense period of eldercare responsibility. Becki had worked at Deloitte and lived in Dallas for seven years when, in 2007, her mother started acting differently. As Becki describes, "She was forgetting things…not remembering where she parked her car or why she was in the grocery store. We knew something was going on. Then, Mom was diagnosed with pancreatic cancer and dementia. She got very sick very quickly."

But rather than drop everything, Becki received her manager's cooperation so she could work remotely. Becki explains: "I worked from Mom's home in Columbus, Ohio, every two weeks. Then I would come home and my brothers would stay there. I worked remotely the whole time." Using a lattice approach, Becki was able to both get her job done and, with the help of a live-in nurse, care for her mother without having to sacrifice one for the other. As a result of her experience, Becki feels a tremendous loyalty to Deloitte, and Deloitte has been able to retain a valuable employee through a trying time.

These stories illustrate that the Corporate Lattice model is a better fit in today's workplace than the century-old corporate ladder, especially since most members of the work force have or will need to care for loved ones either with Alzheimer's or related diseases of the elderly.

1   Interview with Ellen Galinsky by Anne Weisberg on August 24, 2010.

2   Ellen Galinsky, James Bond, et al., *2008 National Study of Employers* (Families and Work Institute, 2008).

3   2010 Sloan Award for When Work Works data from *Families and Work Institute* (received via e-mail on August 24, 2010).

4   Interview with Kathleen Christiansen by Anne Weisberg on August 24, 2010.

*As used in this essay, "Deloitte" means Deloitte LLP and its subsidiaries. Please see www.deloitte.com/us/about for a detailed description of the legal structure of Deloitte LLP and its subsidiaries.

Professional Caregiver

By Doris T., a certified home health aide working on Long Island, New York

I have been a paid caregiver since I was 18. I'm 57 now and work as a certified home health aide. I earn $10 to $12 an hour, depending on the case. This kind of work is about the people. If you don't like people, this isn't the job for you.

It seems to me there are more people with Alzheimer's these days, because people are living longer. Taking care of them means you have to have lots of love and lots of patience. Caring for people with Alzheimer's has taught me all the patience I didn't have when I was younger.

The people I take care of often don't recognize me. So a long time ago, I started giving them my first initial—just D, not Doris. For some reason the D sticks with many of them, and they can remember it.

Every day isn't easy. There are good days and bad days. A good day is when they're in a happy mood. You speak to them, and they respond. You can take them for a walk outside and look at the trees. Some patients still have long-term memories they enjoy, and they will tell you old stories. A family member may let you know if it really happened or if it's just a fantasy.

The hardest times are when a person refuses to eat or be washed. They have lost awareness of themselves and don't know it. You need to convince them that if they don't wash, they will smell. And you have to constantly ask them if they need to go to the toilet. That process can take 30 minutes to an hour. They just don't have a sense of their bodies. Other difficult moments: They don't know the day from the night, and they can wander off.

Recently, I've had a case where the wife takes care of the husband at home. I come every morning Monday through Friday. I get him out of bed, take him to the bathroom, bathe him, shave him and put clean clothes on him. His wife makes him breakfast, and then Senior Services picks him up and takes him to day care. The wife is also getting up in age, so I help her out with some cooking and cleaning. Sometimes I can stay an extra hour, but I have other cases and a family of my own. They are lucky that they can have another aide come in to help for a couple of hours in the evening.

> 66 *I always tell my people with Alzheimer's disease, 'I will see you tomorrow.' I'm trying to let them know that they will be there the next day, and that I will be there for them, too.* 99

This man is a very demanding patient. His wife must love him so much, because she puts up with the behavior. I tell him, "It's nicer when you show your appreciation and say please and thank you." Once in a while he remembers, and then he forgets.

To get by on bad days, I pray for more patience, because you never know if Alzheimer's could happen to you, and you will be the one who needs someone patient to care for you.

I always tell my people with Alzheimer's disease, "I will see you tomorrow." I'm trying to let them know that they will be there the next day, and that I will be there for them, too.

Primary Breadwinner

By Kimberly Davis, an executive with Johnson & Johnson living in Alexandria, Virginia

My husband says he fell in love with me the day I searched the Internet to find a flower-arranging class for his mother. He's always been the Good Son, and like so many African-American men, his mom is his world.

So when he was in his late 20s, and his mother's Alzheimer's disease began to take root, Todd left medical school and moved back to his boyhood home, into his boyhood room, to help his dad care for her. When we started dating a few years later, his family didn't call it Alzheimer's. They called it "memory issues." That was seven years ago.

Todd never finished medical school, and while he makes a good living, it's my salary that pays the mortgage. I struggle daily with my juggling act—primary breadwinner and mother of a toddler. This isn't how I pictured raising a family.

I'm a white-collar professional with some job flexibility, and I do appreciate how fortunate I am compared to most working moms. When my daughter is sick or needs to go to the doctor, I can work from home or go to the office late. I don't get to do story time at the library or visit the neighborhood pool with the other mothers, though. Instead, I cram as much of that in as I can on the weekends and tell myself that it's the quality of the time and not the quantity that's important to my daughter.

Some days I envy the women who have chosen less-demanding careers and are more available to their families. I look at my colleagues with stay-at-home spouses and daydream about how nice it would be if Todd or I could stay home. But we can't, so I try to stay focused on life as it is.

Some days I'm brilliant at work. Other days I do the best I can while worrying about our daughter's allergies or whether we can afford a vacation this year or how to pay for private school some day. I don't hide these thoughts from colleagues or friends, but I also don't talk about them often. As much as I can, I really do try to live in the moment. There's no extra time in my life for complaining.

My husband and I are poster children for the Sandwich Generation, sandwiched between younger and older family members we have to take care of. And some days I resent it. I wish I didn't have to say it's OK for him to take the day off from work to watch his mom so his dad can get some relief. I wish I didn't have to worry every time the phone rings late at night that his mom wandered away from the house and injured herself—again. I wish I didn't have to turn down job opportunities in other parts of the country—places with a lower cost of living and a lifestyle more in keeping with the picture in my head— because I can't imagine asking Todd to leave his mother when she needs him the most. Maybe it sounds selfish, but it's true: I just want it to be easier.

> ❝ *I wish I didn't have to turn down job opportunities in other parts of the country because I can't imagine asking my husband to leave his mother when she needs him the most.* ❞

How do we cope with these challenges? We talk about them. Well, it's not always talking. I pout, I cry, I rage. But at the end of the day I get heard, which is exactly what I need to make it through another day, week, month. I listen to Todd and hear him, too. And this honest communication has brought us closer together.

Ultimately, when I'm frustrated and resentful, I remind myself that I can't begrudge my husband the gift of time he can give to his parents now. It means the world to him. I ask myself how I would feel if the tables were turned. How would I feel if Todd didn't support me doing whatever I felt I needed to do to care for my parents? I know how I'd feel.

So at the same time I'm sharing with you the terrible stresses Alzheimer's places on every member of the family, I also know the underlying truth. And that is what I've always heard people say: "Marry a man who treats his mother well, as he'll likely treat you the same way." With all the trials and the terror and the tears, I know I'm blessed.

Are We Prepared?

What About the Men?

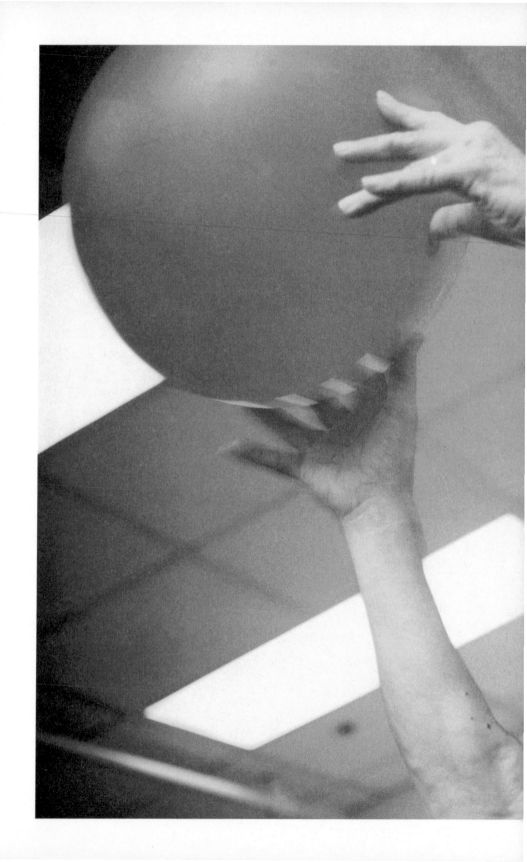

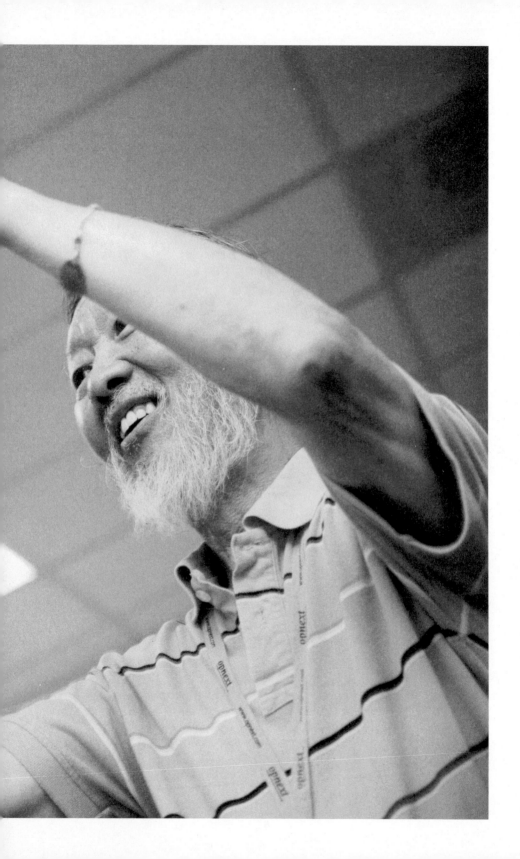

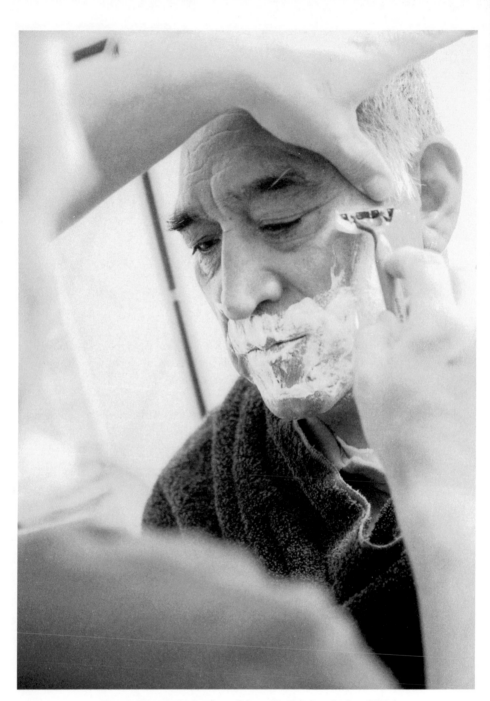

Ricardo Flores, who has been living with Alzheimer's since 2004,
needs help from his son with personal grooming.

What About the Men?

By Michael Kimmel, Ph.D., and Bethany Coston

How do men give—and receive—Alzheimer care? Do they do so differently than women? And, most important, do changes in these differences suggest that men may become more effective and nurturing caregivers and more responsive and receptive patients in the future?

If present trends continue, the 21st century will see many more—perhaps even most— men becoming either a giver or recipient of Alzheimer care. And when they do, they're sure to bump up against traditional notions of masculinity.

For instance, when Ted's wife, Marjorie, was diagnosed with Alzheimer's three years ago at age 73, he was completely unprepared. A 77-year-old retiree, Ted had been slowing down a bit and filled his days with golf and shopping, watching his beloved Padres on television and making toys for their five grandchildren who lived in other states. "I had no idea how to care for Marjorie," he said.

> *What did I know? It was so foreign, like learning another language. I mean, I'm from the generation of men who never changed a diaper for our kids, never cleaned the bathroom, never made the beds. Heck, I can barely fry an egg! But she was losing it— every day, right in front of me, and I had no idea how to care for her. I sort of panicked. I would sometimes go for long drives, so I wouldn't have to be there. I even started drinking a bit. But then I sort of kicked myself in the butt and said to myself, "Ted, you got to play the hand you're dealt." But I won't tell you it hasn't been hard—or that I didn't look at myself, cleaning yet another soiled sheet, and think, "What a wimp you are, man."*

"Harry had always been so fiercely independent," his wife, Linda, said of her 92-year-old husband who'd been diagnosed with Alzheimer's disease four years earlier.

You know, he was the essence of a self-made man. He'd always worked for himself, running his own business, being the family chauffeur, an equal partner in the kitchen. But as his disease progressed, I could see that sense of autonomy and the pride he took in being so independent slowly eroding. He'd deny it, of course. Try to fight through it. Pretend he understood when he didn't, that he recognized people or remembered events when I knew he didn't. I played along, trying to affirm that sense of himself, even as I knew we couldn't sustain the charade. Gradually, we couldn't anymore. He left the stove on a couple of times, and I became afraid he could hurt himself, or just get hurt, or even burn the house down.

Once when I was cooking dinner, I grumbled that I needed a tomato. Harry said, "I'll get it honey," and after I protested, he walked to the store. He came back with a potato. I tried not to get angry—he seemed so pleased with himself for running the errand. I said, "A tomato, not a potato." He looked so embarrassed, sheepish, like a little boy who had displeased his mother. "I'll go get it," he said. "I promise." How could I not let him go? I wrote "1 tomato" on a piece of note paper and sent him back to the store, only a block or two away. He came back 20 minutes later and triumphantly presented me with another potato. The note paper was crumpled into a ball in his pocket. He said he had looked at it but couldn't really remember what it was for.

Ted and Harry represent two sides of the Alzheimer male equation: caregiver and patient. Caregiving and being cared for know no gender. Both women and men are capable of caregiving, and both certainly may be in need of care. And yet caregiving, and being cared for, are among the most gendered activities in which we engage. Both giving and receiving care is seen as feminine. Caring is an expression of what is often perceived as a "natural" femininity, an extension of women's biological and evolutionary imperative to care for the young. Caring requires emotional resources as well as various skills, and these emotional resources—patience, calm, nurturance—have, rightly or wrongly, long been coded as "feminine."

Women the likely caregivers

As earlier studies have shown, women are more likely to be caregivers, and they make more substantial sacrifices for the role. In 2010, of the 11.2 million people caring specifically for people with Alzheimer's and dementia, 6.7 million, or about 60 percent are women. Female caregivers provide more hours of care and a higher level of care than male caregivers. For example, the new Alzheimer's Association 2010 Women and Alzheimer's poll shows half of women caregivers and a third of men caregivers are providing more than 40 hours per week of care.

Another study shows women spend an average of four hours more caregiving per week than men (24 hours for women vs. 18 hours for men), and female caregivers are more likely than males to help with the personal activities of getting dressed (47 percent vs. 28 percent respectively), bathing or showering (37 percent vs. 18 percent) and dealing with incontinence or adult undergarments (36 percent vs. 23 percent). Moreover, over half of female caregivers of people with Alzheimer's and other dementias are employed, mostly full-time; and 50 percent said they did not have a choice in accepting responsibility for providing Alzheimer care.[1]

The tenets of masculinity

The acceptance of the role of "patient" also varies between men and women. Elderly, disabled and ill relatives rely on the labor of family, with between 50 and 75 percent of all care recipients needing help not only with difficult tasks, such as preparing meals, cleaning the house or managing finances, but also menial ones such as dressing, eating and going to the bathroom.[2] Being cared for is seen as feminine. To require this kind of care is to be dependent, vulnerable and permeable, contradicting the very tenets of masculinity. This likely accounts for the higher levels of acting out—swearing, yelling, falling down, making excessive demands and the like—as well as males' lower levels of helping behaviors, such as giving praise and helping with caring chores/tasks.[3]

> More men caregivers than women think that caregiving for someone with Alzheimer's puts a strain on their marriage.

Masculinity varies with both time and place, creating a multitude of masculinities. However, generally, a dominant model exists—a "hegemonic" definition of masculinity, to which men are expected to adhere.[4] In the United States, the dominant image of masculinity that emerged in the 19th century was "the self-made man."[5] Known generally for manly stoicism and fierce resolve, he was emotionally impenetrable, an armor-plated machine who showed no weakness. In the mid-1970s, psychologists created a masculinity scale that codified these traits.[6] Brannon defined these as the four basic "rules" of manhood:

1. "No Sissy Stuff": Manhood is defined by distance from what was perceived as feminine.

2. "Be a Big Wheel": Manhood is measured by the size of one's paycheck; wealth, power, status and success are its defining features.

3. "Be a Sturdy Oak": Manly stoicism is what makes men reliable in a crisis.

4. "Give 'Em Hell": Men are adventuresome, exhibiting risk-taking and aggression.[7]

More recently, Kilmartin broke these down into 12 distinctive personality traits: strength, independence, achievement, hard working, dominance, heterosexuality, toughness, aggressiveness, unemotional, physical, competitiveness and forcefulness.[8]

This traditional definition of masculinity retains a powerful influence over what both men and women believe men should be. Moreover, psychologists argue that gender conformity is both unattainable and internally contradictory, and men who cannot conform appropriately feel adherence to the role is a strain.[9] Even men who succeed feel the strain in doing so, and the harmful components of the role present problems.[10]

Masculinity and males with Alzheimer's

Being a patient contradicts the definition of manhood, leaving a person vulnerable, weakened and dependent. As a result, many men resist seeking health care. Men pay far less attention to diet and substance abuse than women, and they perform self-exams and seek preventive screenings less often as well. Why? As health researcher Will Courtenay writes:

> A man who does gender correctly would be relatively unconcerned about his health and well-being in general. He would see himself as stronger, both physically and emotionally than most women. He would think of himself as independent, not needing to be nurtured by others. He would be unlikely to ask others for help ... He would face danger fearlessly, take risks frequently, and have little concern for his own safety."[11]

Or, as one Zimbabwean man put it to an interviewer, "Real men don't get sick."[12]

The Alzheimer's Association Women and Alzheimer's poll shows a stark gap in the responses of men and women caring for someone with Alzheimer's when asked if they themselves fear developing the disease. Two-thirds of women report they are frightened of developing Alzheimer's; nearly 60 percent of men state they are not. This feeling and acknowledging of health-related vulnerability and fear is one of the largest gender gaps of the poll.

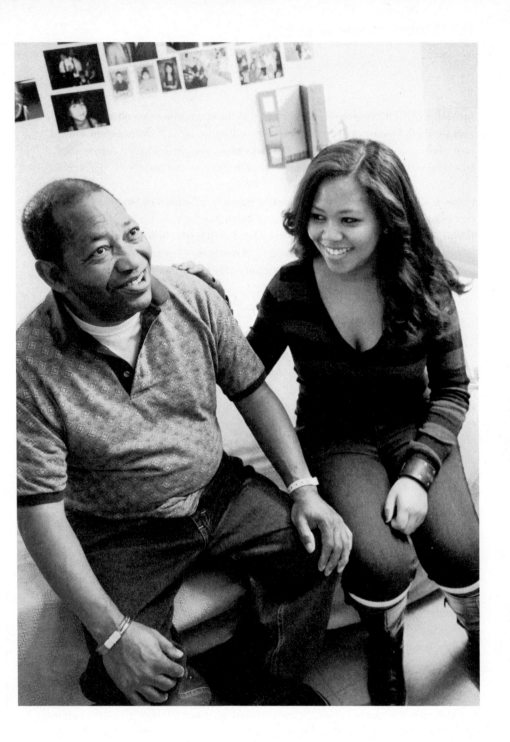

Avoidance of health care could also be related to the often demeaning nature of the visit—it's cold, you're naked and the doctor is talking to you as if you're a child. Others, even, see it as a waste of money—perhaps why more men are uninsured than women. One New Yorker summed it up as the "What I don't know can't hurt me" approach.

However, the very requirements that make a man a "real" man may be the very things that endanger his health. The four causes of death that have the highest differential by sex are the four illnesses most closely associated with gender behavior, not biological sex: accidents, suicide, cirrhosis (drinking) and homicide.[13] A researcher once suggested creating a warning label: "Caution: Masculinity May Be Hazardous to Your Health."

More men (53 percent) than women (45 percent) report coordinating their schedules, duties and responsibilities at least daily with their wives.

Alzheimer's can be experienced by men as emasculating: the mind's gradual diminishment may be experienced as a loss of manhood. Caregivers, both male and female, need to be aware of the ways that succumbing to Alzheimer's—indeed, developing the disease in the first place—can be experienced as gender non-conforming and that some male patients will attempt to compensate for their perceived loss of manhood by emphasizing other dimensions of that traditional role.

For example, the strain on gender identity experienced by male care recipients may be the source of some gender differences in patient behavior. Research suggests that males with Alzheimer's are more likely to act out and less likely to help their caregivers. Care recipients' problematic behaviors have been studied extensively and are consistently found to be influential predictors of caregiver distress.[14] Such problems (e.g., falling down, making excessive demands or asking repetitive questions) are typically associated with either physical illness or cognitive impairment.[15] A recent study discovered that wife-caregivers reported a higher incidence of problem behaviors among their care-receiving male spouses.[16]

When normal routine activities are compromised, as they are with the onset of Alzheimer's disease, some men may feel a corresponding erosion of their masculine self, their sense of manly autonomy and self-control. In one study, over half (52 percent) of care recipients had difficulty in carrying out three or more activities of daily living

Table 1: Top Functional Problems of Alzheimer Care Recipients
and the Percent Reporting Problem in Previous Week

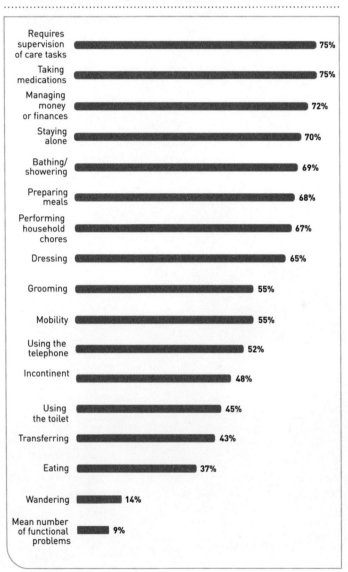

Requires supervision of care tasks	75%
Taking medications	75%
Managing money or finances	72%
Staying alone	70%
Bathing/ showering	69%
Preparing meals	68%
Performing household chores	67%
Dressing	65%
Grooming	55%
Mobility	55%
Using the telephone	52%
Incontinent	48%
Using the toilet	45%
Transferring	43%
Eating	37%
Wandering	14%
Mean number of functional problems	9%

Source: California CRC Uniform Assessment Database, 2001, N=3,476.

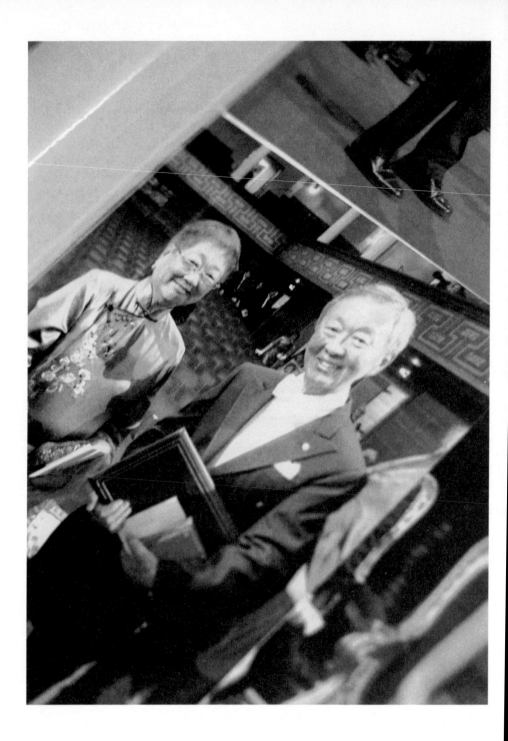

such as bathing, dressing and eating. Nearly nine out of ten (89 percent) reported difficulty with one or more instrumental activities of daily living (e.g., preparing meals, using the telephone, managing money and taking medications (see Table 1).

Alzheimer's may be especially difficult to reconcile with traditional notions of masculinity that stress autonomy and control, because these are often gradually eroded by the disease. Problem behaviors—falling down, questioning, excessive demands, cursing, yelling, etc.—were a significant causal factor in caregiving wives' rates of reported depression. Moreover, husbands' problem behaviors can be a significant predictor of wives' maladaptation to caregiving.[17] That is, wife-caregivers whose husbands exhibited problem behaviors were likely to feel distant from their husbands and burdened by caregiving.

Masculinity and the male Alzheimer caregiver

The same things that make a male patient feel emasculated often make being a male caregiver stressful. It can be difficult to incorporate the role responsibilities into the traditional definitions of masculinity. However, it's important to remember that just because men may perform caregiving differently than women doesn't necessarily mean they do it worse.

Male caregivers, for example, tend to believe that they can simply "add" caregiving to their list of other activities. Male caregivers are more likely to be working full-time (60 percent) than female caregivers (41 percent), and female caregivers are more likely to be working part-time (14 percent) than male caregivers (6 percent). However, this could be because women are more likely than men to have decreased their hours, passed up promotions or assignments, taken leaves of absence, switched their employment from full- to part-time, quit jobs or retired early because of their caregiving role.

In another study, conformity to traditional masculinity was actually associated with having greater perceived competence at caregiving.[18] After all, while caring may be gender-nonconforming, being good at what you do (competence) may be an even stronger gendered trait.

However, it's equally clear that such an additive model of caregiving, in which the caregiver simply adds the caregiving duties to an otherwise long list of gender-conforming activities, can also be quite stressful. A California study found that being a caregiver for someone with Alzheimer's is associated with increased risk for cardiovascular disease, especially for males.[19]

Traditional masculinity ill prepares men for caregiving. However, husbands may feel less depression than women in caregiving positions because the men receive help from their wives in the caregiving process. Miller reported that female care recipients provided their caregiving spouses with several forms of support, which included helping with chores, providing companionship and making them feel useful.[20] These helping behaviors can lessen the stress of caregiving. Indeed, Kaye and Appelgate found that male caregivers in general described emotional gratification an important motivation for caregiving, although many also reported that they ascribed to themselves many affective traits associated with femininity.[21]

However, caring for people with Alzheimer's is often tedious and time-consuming. One study found that caregivers of people with Alzheimer's provide an average of 14 more hours of care than those of other physically impaired individuals.[22] This extra time is probably accounted for by the extra care patients need, specifically companionship care, i.e., supervision for safety. Many people with Alzheimer's get angry and frustrated easily, and engage in problem behaviors more frequently than other types of patients (whether by choice or otherwise). Unlike other patients, those with Alzheimer's are also less likely to be able to help their caregivers, resulting in a greater amount of stress/strain on the caregiver.

Overall, it seems as though women caregivers are more greatly affected psychologically and physically by caring for someone with Alzheimer's.[23] However, we must keep in mind that the tenets of masculinity call for stoicism and emotionlessness, both of which would lead men to underreport or not report their feelings of stress, depression or pain from the job.

Caring and receiving care in the 21st century

Caregiving is not an "identity," something you are, but rather a set of practices, something you "do." While gender shapes our experiences of both the giving and the receiving of care, it is equally true that anyone—male or female—can be an effective caregiver. In fact, in the past two decades, men have increased the amount of time they spend in caregiving with their young children enormously. Men now spend as much time with children in 2010 as women did in 1980. (Women have also increased their time.)

Men have increased their caregiving with children at little cost to their sense of themselves as men. And if men can do it with their children, it's possible that they can also become more active and involved with their parents. And if that is possible, then it is even possible that they can receive care in ways they had not previously.

The current cohorts of both men with Alzheimer's and male caregivers are also from an earlier era, likely born before the advent of the gender revolution of the 1960s. More likely to subscribe to more traditional gender identities, this is a generation that may be inhibited by the gender roles of the past. They are men like Harry, who prided himself on his autonomy and independence in the public sphere, and men like Ted, who seemed equally proud of his "dependence" in the private sphere—that is, his learned helplessness, his inability to take care of himself as a badge of masculinity.

Younger cohorts of men are more egalitarian at home and at work. They are as accustomed to female colleagues and co-workers as they are competent at cooking and cleaning. As these men age, the traditional ideologies to which their fathers and grandfathers subscribed will be, at least partly, supplanted by a masculinity of nurturance, caregiving and love. And they will feel no less manly for it.

ENDNOTES

1 Unpublished data from the NAC/AARP survey of caregiving in the United States, prepared under contract for the Alzheimer's Association by Matthew Greenwald and Associates, April 8, 2010.

2 The MetLife Study of Alzheimer's Disease: The Caregiving Experience. August 2006. MetLife Mature Market Institute in conjunction with LifePlans, Inc.

3 J. Wider, "Alzheimer's Cases Expected to Skyrocket Over the Next 50 Years," Society for Women's Health Research, 2003.

4 R.W. Connell, 1992. "A very straight gay: Masculinity, homosexual experience, and the dynamics of gender," *American Sociological Review* 57 (6):735-75, 1992.———. 1994. "Gender and power," *Different roles, different voices: women and politics in the United States and Europe:* 268; Connell and J.W. Messerschmidt; "Hegemonic masculinity: Rethinking the concept," *Gender & Society* 19 (6):829, 2005

5 M. Kimmel, 1996, *Manhood in America: A Cultural History.* New York: Free Press.

6 J.M. O'Neil, 1981, "Male sex role conflicts, sexism, and masculinity: Psychological implications for men, women, and the counseling psychologist," *The Counseling Psychologist* 9 (2):61.

7 R. Brannon, 1976, "The male sex role: Our culture's blueprint of manhood, and what it's done for us lately," *The forty-nine percent majority: The male sex role,* 1–48.

8 C. Kilmartin and C.T. Kilmartin, 2000. *The masculine self.* McGraw-Hill Higher Education.

9 J.H. Pleck, 1981. *The myth of masculinity.* Cambridge, MA: MIT Press.

10 J.R. Mahalik, B.D. Locke, H. Theodore, R.J. Cournoyer and B.F. Lloyd, 2001, "A cross-national and cross-sectional comparison of men's gender role conflict and its relationship to social intimacy and self-esteem," *Sex Roles* 45 (1):1-14; J.M. Robertson, A.L. Johnson, S.L. Benton, B.A. Janey, J. Cabral and

J.A. Woodford, 2002. "What's in a picture? Comparing gender constructs of younger and older adults," *The Journal of Men's Studies* 11 (1):1-27.

11 W.H. Courtenay, 1998, "Better to die than cry? A longitudinal and constructionist study of masculinity and the health risk behaviour of young American men," *University of California at Berkeley.* Dissertation Abstracts International, 59(08A), (Publication number 9902042).

12 J. Cohen, 2010. "Men Likely to Put Off Doctor: Men Avoid Preventative Health Care in Sickness and in Health," ABC News, http://abcnews.go.com/Health/story?id=116898&page=1; M. Foreman, 1999, "AIDS and men: taking risks or taking responsibility?" *Zed Books.*

13 See also Broom and Cavenagh, 2010.

14 M. Pinquart, and S. Sorensen, 2003, "Differences between caregivers and noncaregivers in psychological health and physical health: A meta-analysis," *Psychology and Aging* 18 (2):250-267; R. Schulz, A.T. O'Brien, J. Bookwala and K. Fleissner, 1995, "Psychiatric and physical morbidity effects of dementia caregiving: Prevalence, correlates, and causes," *The Gerontologist* 35 (6):771.

15 J. Bookwala and R Schulz, 2000, "A Comparison of Primary Stressors, Secondary Stressors, and Depressive Symptoms Between Elderly Caregiving Husbands and Wives* 1: The Caregiver Health Effects Study," *Psychology and Aging* 15 (4):607-616.

16 Ibid.

17 M.M. Seltzer and LW Li, 1996, "The transitions of caregiving: Subjective and objective definitions," *The Gerontologist* 36 (5):614.

18 Wilkin, 1996.

19 Mills, et al., 2009.

20 B. Miller, 1990. "Gender differences in spouse caregiver strain: Socialization and role explanations," *Journal of Marriage and the Family* 52 (2):311-321.

21 Kaye and Applegate, 2010.

22 The MetLife Study of Alzheimer's Disease: The Caregiving Experience, August 2006, MetLife Mature Market Institute in conjunction with LifePlans, Inc.

23 Unpublished data from the NAC/AARP survey of caregiving in the United States, prepared under contract for the Alzheimer's Association by Matthew Greenwald and Associates, April 8, 2010.

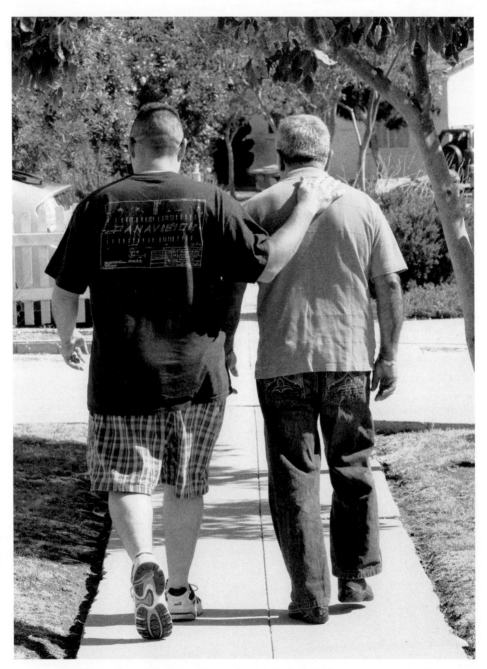

Arturo Flores gives his father a hand while taking a walk. Father and son have not let Ricardo's diagnosis of Alzheimer's disease inhibit their spending time together.

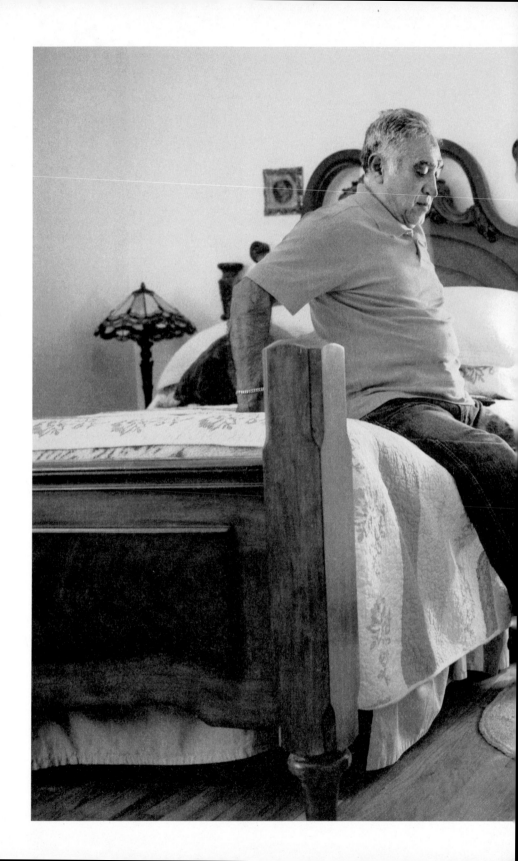

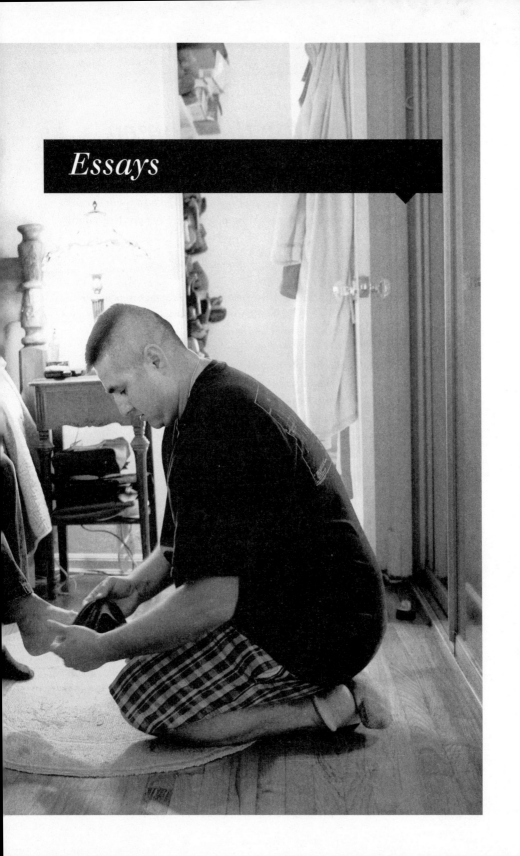

Essays

Caring for the Women in Their Lives

By Jamal Simmons, political commentator and campaign media adviser who contributed to The Shriver Report: A Woman's Nation Changes Everything

Last year, I attended a beautiful and heartwarming recommitment ceremony for the grandparents of a friend. Sixty-three years after first committing to be there for each other in sickness and health, the sickness was here.

After raising two children, adoring four granddaughters and having a life filled with friends and service to the community, they were coping with the wife's advancing Alzheimer's disease. The husband was her primary caregiver, making her meals, choosing her clothes, administering her medication and managing the family team caring for their matriarch. Knowing how uncertain his wife felt about the future, he planned the recommitment ceremony to let her know, while she could still appreciate it, that he would always be there for her.

Men sometimes get a bad rap in the caregiving department, but today a third of unpaid caregivers are men looking after a wife, mother, grandmother, aunt or friend with Alzheimer's, and they can be incredibly dutiful at it. A friend told me her parents had been divorced for 30 years, but that didn't stop her father from providing daily care when her mom was diagnosed and went to a long-term care facility. She said, "Daddy had breakfast with her each day, washed her clothes and met with Mom's medical team with my sister."

The nature of men's caregiving is all over the map. One geriatric care professional told me she found that older men who came of age in a world of more traditional gender roles could be especially unprepared for monitoring medical regimens, shopping for groceries, preparing meals and other tasks caregivers provide people with Alzheimer's. Often these men, many of whom served in the military, try to tough it out until others intervene when it becomes clear they need help. This is in contrast to sons and grandsons of people with Alzheimer's, who she finds tend to be more willing to seek help from other relatives or healthcare professionals. Indeed, almost half of all caregivers do.

Alzheimer's Association research reveals that children and grandchildren tend to be the vast majority of caretakers, but for many men, bathing mom or grandma or taking her to the bathroom may simply be too intimate a task to manage. Others, still in the midst of their careers or acting as the primary family breadwinners, find it incredibly difficult to supply the level of attention people with Alzheimer's require.

> 66 *Many men who meet the challenge of caring for someone with Alzheimer's also speak of great rewards and comfort.* 99

Taking care of someone with Alzheimer's can be incredibly difficult for any caregiver, and each man who always had a mom or wife to care for him takes to the role reversal differently. But while the demands and pains can be great, many men who meet the challenge of caring for a person with the disease also speak of great rewards and comfort.

My own dad, who spent more than a year caring daily for my grandmother while she was hospitalized for a non-Alzheimer-related illness, offers another perspective. As a pastor, he has observed that men who have played a greater role in child rearing, which often requires many of the same duties, are better equipped to take care of their parents. It impacts your life, he says, in much the same way.

Sadly, my friend's grandmother passed away just a few months after that lovely recommitment ceremony. At her funeral, their minister stood at the lectern and reminded the husband of his wife's fear of being alone. Now there would be days the husband felt lonely, the minister told him sympathetically. On those days he should take comfort, because those feelings of loneliness were his final act of loving sacrifice for his wife, who never had to be alone at the end.

"She Walked Through the Looking Glass"

By Barry Petersen, a CBS News correspondent based in Denver and author of
Jan's Story: Love Lost to the Long Goodbye of Alzheimer's

*I*t happened on a balmy Tokyo summer weekend in 2005. I went to work that Saturday morning to prepare a story about robots for my job as the CBS News correspondent covering Asia. When I came home that afternoon, Jan had walked through the looking glass, and she stayed there for three days.

During those three days she heard voices in our apartment telling her people were coming to dinner and other voices at the grocery store telling her what to buy. She was making sentences with all the correct words, but they were out of order. The second evening, she dressed in layers of street clothes and crawled into bed. The third, she put hamburgers in a pot for boiling water, put a frying pan on top, turned the burner to max and went to sleep.

On the fourth day, Jan woke up seemingly fine, with no memory of what had happened. She was 55, and those three days were a peek into the future for me.

It was 4 a.m. Tokyo time when I finally reached a San Francisco neurologist and described the symptoms: "From what you say, she has early-onset Alzheimer's disease."

When did it start? There had been clues I'd missed. Jan had been repeating herself, and she rarely left the house on her own. She wasn't herself—a bright, vivacious woman who had been a successful Seattle TV anchor before we got married on Valentine's Day 20 years before. We called each other Darling and Darling. CBS News sent us to Tokyo, Moscow, London and now back to Asia, with apartments in Tokyo and Beijing. We joked that we'd someday chase each other around in wheelchairs at the old folks' home. But now Alzheimer's was making me her caregiver.

Like most men, I always believed your decency and self-worth come from providing for and protecting the people you love—in my case, Jan, my daughters from my first marriage, my granddaughter. Men also approach problems by coming up with a strategy, an action plan, a solution. We must Do Something. Somehow I thought I'd be able to beat back a disease that is 100 percent terminal.

At first, I congratulated myself that I had it under control. I phoned Jan during the day, making sure she wasn't leaving the stove on. I covered for her as she faded, like gently suggesting a favorite dish at a restaurant, when I realized she couldn't understand the menu anymore.

But my action plan slowly crumbled as the disease crept forward and took more of Jan away.

I remember the first time she forgot me. It was in Beijing. "You have a wedding ring," she said. "Are you married?" That hurt, but when she rearranged her medication schedule while I was gone on a trip for work, I knew she needed more help. I hired a retired nurse from Tacoma, Washington, to come to Tokyo as our live-in caregiver. I was taking care of business.

Men don't always acknowledge how much they get from the woman in their lives. For me, being with Jan was the core of my own strength. Her support and love were a well I could always draw from when I ran dry. Now, the support was fading away, and I was power-less to do anything about it. I pushed away self-doubt and loneliness with anger. I know I became hard to be around, to work with. I consoled myself with food and drink.

The caretaking scenario I'd set up lasted less than a year. First came Jan's explosive anger: clenched fist, red face, spitting, sputtering anger. She became furious that, she claimed, four women, including the caregiver, were in the house eating all our food. She would storm out of the apartment and show up at my office in a fury. She threw tan-trums in stores, on the train. She'd lock herself in a room for hours. I believe she was furious at what was happening to her, how much of her life and independence she was losing. More and more of her slipped away. And more and more of me was buckling under the stress.

The caregiver said it was time to move Jan into an assisted living facility in the United States. Plenty of people said I was abandoning ship, abandoning Jan. Others realized I was trying to save her—and also myself.

As I walked away from the facility in May 2008, under an unexpectedly sunny Seattle sky, I realized that this was the end of Jan and Barry, the end of Darling and Darling. I couldn't protect her from what Alzheimer's did to her, and all the love I was capable of giving couldn't stop it or even ease it. That's when I learned how a man can fall to the ground because he's weeping so hard—from guilt, from sadness, from love, from loss.

I've written a book, *Jan's Story*, to share our experiences. I don't know what I expected, but I've been surprised some of the strongest reactions to it come from men whose own spouses have Alzheimer's. Some are still caregiving, some have placed their wives as I did, and some are dealing with the sadness of death.

> **❝ We're blindsided when Alzheimer's steals our wives. If we let ourselves feel it, Alzheimer's is also stealing the structure upon which we build our self-worth. ❞**

Why the deepest, most gut-wrenching reactions from men? Because as shocking as the Alzheimer diagnosis is to any family, men are totally blindsided by the disease in their wives. It shakes who they are to the core. Men fool themselves into believing they can handle such a thing. While we so casually tell our women, "I'd be lost without you," we are really unprepared to learn what that means.

What Alzheimer's steals away from us is a friend like no other—a friend who isn't another male, because men compete with other men. Our only friend who draws out our feelings when we hide them, which is often. A friend with whom we share that physical contact—that kiss, that touch—we sometimes can't admit we need. A man's wife gives him reasons to feel good about himself that no one else can provide—when he buys her presents, when he bursts with pride because she's on his arm, when he watches with pleasure and awe as she shapes a career or a family or—how does she do it?—both.

It's a cliché only because it's so true: Women complete us, and men don't always like to admit it. On the outside, we prefer to measure success by money, career, status, even cars. We forget that it's so often our partner who creates the circle within which we can flourish, within which we become the men we are meant to be.

That's why we're blindsided when Alzheimer's steals our wives. If we let ourselves feel it, Alzheimer's is also stealing the structure upon which we build our self-worth. When it takes away our support, we realize how much we weren't standing on our own. She was the one we needed most to survive this journey.

So now, the long goodbye continues. There is plenty of practical caregiving advice out there. But who can tell us if we're doing it right for the woman we love? Only she could, but she no longer can.

I left Asia, resettled in Denver and moved Jan from Seattle to a facility a few minutes from where I live. I go see her, but she no longer sees me. She doesn't remember what she did a minute earlier. She often chatters away in sentences no one can understand.

One day not too long ago on a visit, Jan smiled and said sweetly, "Will you marry me?" I couldn't tell her that we've been married for 25 years. She wouldn't understand. It hurt.

But thinking about it later, there was sweetness that she still found me a person she could marry. I cried and vowed to preserve the memory of that lovely moment. And I would preserve it for both of us, because for Jan, that memory is long since gone.

Role Reversal:
A Son Caring for His Mother

By 56-year-old Randy Sibbett of Sacramento, California, who moved with his new wife back into his childhood home so he could take care of his mother with Alzheimer's

My father died two years ago, seven years after my mother was diagnosed with Alzheimer's disease. He was her primary caregiver. Back then, I didn't fully realize the connection between Mom's Alzheimer's and Dad's own health, as he had heart troubles anyway. I've since learned that, in fact, elderly spousal caregivers suffer an increased risk for illness themselves and a higher rate of mortality, and they often die before their loved ones do. But now I think back on the many times Dad talked of his sorrow and stress as he watched his bride of 67 years mentally fading away from him.

I made a promise to my father on his deathbed that Mom would remain in our family home they bought back in 1954, just a few months before my first birthday. So I moved back in with my wife, and I'm now my mom's primary caregiver. And today, I fully understand what the sorrow and stress of caregiving can do to you.

> 66 *Her illness has required that I take on the role of nurturer. This character trait is unnatural for men, as we're born and raised to be providers and protectors.* 99

Before Dad died, Mom had already lost the ability to help around the house. She couldn't remember where the dishes, silverware, pots and pans went, let alone how to pay the bills, which she had always done. Dad had to take away her driver's license because she couldn't remember how to take trips she had made so many times before, such as to the hairdresser and back.

In the two years since Dad's death, Mom has become unable to do just about everything else. She is incapable of making any decisions on her own—for example, what to wear or what to order at a restaurant. Where she used to get angry Dad had taken her license away, now she says she just wishes she knew how to drive, forgetting she ever knew how.

When people ask, "How is your mom doing?" I explain, "She is growing younger." What I mean is that compared to a child, who grows older (more independent), my mother is growing younger (more dependent).

Her illness has required that I take on the role of nurturer. This character trait is unnatural for men, as we're born and raised to be providers and protectors. Nurturing her means I've had to learn extraordinary, even unimaginable, amounts of compassion and self-control. I've learned how to extend patience and grace to Mom even in times where patience and grace feel beyond me.

So far, the most difficult thing for me is dealing with the times when she's incontinent. Urinary incontinence isn't so bad; it's the bowel incontinence that tests me the most. When she disappears into the bathroom and does not come out for an extended period of time, that is the signal that something is wrong. She is too proud and embarrassed to call for help, so she tries to take care of the situation herself. Of course, that makes the mess worse and more difficult for me because now I have to clean both her and the bathroom. Who on earth could ever have imagined the day would come when I would be changing the diapers of the woman who changed mine?

I've also had to realize that someone with Alzheimer's is incapable of learning, incapable of adjusting and incapable of prolonged rational thought. For them, it doesn't matter how many times they've heard something or said something or done something. I've had to accept the fact that "Every time is the first time!" At meals, she remarks how good something tastes each and every time she puts a bite of it into her mouth. She reads today's mail aloud over and over and over again. The dog is getting fat because she can't remember she already gave him a cookie a few minutes ago.

There are other ways caregiving doesn't come naturally to me. I'm a single-focus, task-oriented person. Having the day broken into pieces by the constant stream of chores and emergencies and demands of caregiving is difficult for me. Starting, stopping and then starting again is not my forte. I lose my concentration and often lose track of priorities.

Caregiving is isolating, too. I've had to accept that it is not just Mom who is housebound, but me as well. It's so difficult to get time off to recharge your batteries. She can't be left alone for any period of time without a respite caregiver. We've called on seven differ-

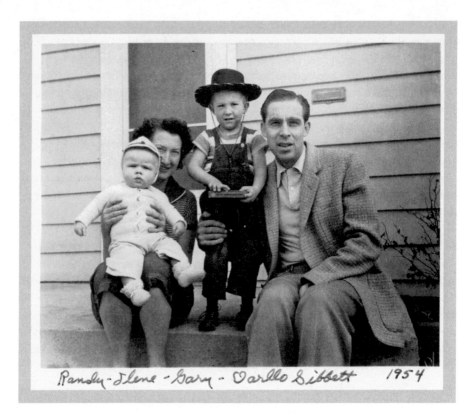

Randy - Ilene - Gary - Orville Sibbett   1954

ent respite caregivers, but bringing in someone new and making them familiar with the surroundings and every nuance of our caregiving routine takes time and, once again, patience. On several occasions, respite caregivers have broken their commitments at the last moment, requiring us to cancel an evening out, a day off, a weekend getaway or a vacation.

I realize that what truly hurts the most is that there is no such thing as a meaningful conversation with my mother anymore. In some respects, it feels like I have already lost both parents.

> **66 I hope and pray that when Mom's time on this earth is concluded, she feels I did as good a job taking care of her in her twilight years as she did taking care of me growing up. 99**

But it's also an honor to take care of my mom at this juncture in our lives. I rely on my faith, knowing that all things are for His glory. My wife, Mary, who—believe it or not!—is a manager for the California Department of Aging, is, next to the Lord, my rock. I'm so fortunate that Mary has been Mom's greatest advocate with medical professionals, respite caregivers and government agencies.

Yes, at times caring for my mom is a struggle, but I know two things for sure. There are lessons to be learned through this experience, and the path I'm on today is leading me somewhere I'm supposed to go. I hope and pray that when Mom's time on this earth is concluded, she feels I did as good a job taking care of her in her twilight years as she did taking care of me growing up.

"Your Mom's Not What She Was"

By Chris Matthews, host of MSNBC's Hardball with Chris Matthews *and* The Chris Matthews Show *on NBC*

*W*e found the paper with Mom's scribbled writing. She had been trying one last time, I imagine, to write something intelligible. But she couldn't even get through the first sentence.

It must be excruciating to realize you have Alzheimer's disease.

Think about what it takes to cook a big meal for seven people each night. Timing is everything. The pot roast, turkey or ham has to be in the oven the right amount of time. The vegetables need to be done at the same moment. In families like ours back then, people were ready to sit down to eat precisely at 6 o'clock. Any later, and we'd start to wonder, "Where's dinner? What's wrong?"

For decades, Mom gave us the grandest meals she could, while staying within her budget. She never took shortcuts. She baked a cake practically every day, giving us each a slice for dessert after supper, then another for a bedtime snack. That's the kind of mom she was.

So when you lose the ability to do all this—to perfectly prepare and time an elaborate meal each evening—you know you're losing something vital, something of yourself. When Mom began to show symptoms of Alzheimer's, that's exactly what happened. She couldn't prepare a meal anymore—because, to her distress, she just couldn't tell time.

"Your mom's not what she was," Dad said to me one day.

That was how it began for our family—the decade-long decline that went pretty much by the book. Mom was behaving in ways that followed the usual course for someone with the disease.

"Classic," Dad would say, having read up on the clinical descriptions of Alzheimer's. It's good that he did, otherwise he might have taken it personally when Mom, in her confusion, blamed him. He knew it was the disease. He knew he was sharing the experience of Alzheimer caregivers everywhere.

"Classic." That was his way of coping. If you asked him how Mom was doing, that would be his answer every time.

My mother had always been a fighter. She fought to get us everything: the best schools, piano lessons, a house at the shore in summer, college, everything. Our hopes were her pride.

> 66 *With each passing visit, children return home to see their parent changed. And the changes are so great, they can forget the parent they once knew so well.* 99

But by the time all our hopes and dreams had come true and she could have enjoyed the success of her kids, she had lost even the ability to tell time.

Alzheimer's is indeed the long goodbye. With each passing visit, children return home to see their parent changed. And the changes are so great, they can forget the parent they once knew so well. Old memories can get wiped away in the presence of one who has no memory. As the warmth and joy of the past recedes and fades, the tragedy looms and grows. Only by reading the hopeful, caring letters she wrote to me in college and later in the Peace Corps, can I still find the Mom I remember.

When our mother died, all of us were too devastated to speak—all but my brother, Bruce. He gathered himself, stood up and went to the altar on behalf of his brothers and Dad to speak for Mom.

With a strong voice overpowering his emotion, he said, "Mom would speak for us."

Today, I know we all need to speak out. We need to do all we can to end this disease. Mom would have done it for us.

Facing This Demon
Called Alzheimer's

By Larry Butcher, board member and past chair of Alzheimer's Community Care, past chair of Florida's Alzheimer's Disease Advisory Committee and retired marketing consultant

*J*eannette, my wife of more than 50 years, died last year from the ravages of Alzheimer's disease. She was a vibrant, loving woman who thrived on motherhood, family, friends and community service. For 17 years, this disease took its terrible toll on all of us.

When Alzheimer's started to possess Jeannette, I went into deep denial. I kept my feelings hidden not just from everyone else, but from myself, too. Powering ahead had always been my way. My whole life, my guiding principle had been to deal with challenges head-on. In fact, I would have disdain for others who didn't face up to the trials in their lives with faith and their eyes open.

But I couldn't face this. I couldn't even say the words "Alzheimer's disease" out loud. When it took away Jeannette's spirit and her magnificent smile, I kept my pain and anguish about what the disease was doing to her and to us as a couple deep within me, until it made me sick. I became angry and chronically depressed.

As my mental and physical health deteriorated, my spirit was tested. Only then, at the lowest ebb of my life, did I realize that for the sake of my boys, my parents and myself, I needed to face this demon called Alzheimer's and reach out to others for help.

I spoke with my pastor, who comforted me by affirming that I had the strength to recover and heal myself through faith. Then I went into action. My research led me to a true friend and resource for caregivers and families, Alzheimer's Community Care.

There I did something I would never have done before in my life. I started to attend the kind of support groups I had always thought of as "griping gatherings." I soon learned that you only get out of such an experience how much you put into it.

I realized I had a choice. If I were going to continue to be a son to my mom and dad, a father to my sons, a grandfather, and a dedicated caregiver to someone who needed me to be more than just a husband, I had to proceed on the strength of my faith. That was the choice I had to make, and I am glad I did. I got fully engaged in support group discussions, exposing myself to others who were also suffering and in great pain. And that is exactly how I started to heal from my grief and despair.

I became a support group leader and eventually joined the board of Alzheimer's Community Care. Later, I was appointed to a state advisory committee on Alzheimer's disease. Eventually, I had the good fortune to chair both of those organizations.

I would never have discovered the true strength of faith, the strength of family, the strength of community-based organizations and the strength of a marriage where you give 100 percent and expect nothing in return if I had not become the dedicated caregiver Jeannette needed.

Jeannette has been gone more than a year, and now I am traveling the United States, seeing beautiful parts of this great country of ours, doing missionary work for my church. I have a new purpose and a new lease on life. It's a life I would never have had without the help of Alzheimer's Community Care, my parents, my sons, my community and my faith.

How fortunate I am to have been able to reach out during the darkest days of my life and come to the realization that the greatest love I could give my Jeannette was to be her compassionate, loyal and committed caregiver and to "grow where I was planted."

"She Was the Love of My Life"

*By Terrell Owens, wide receiver for the National Football League's
Cincinnati Bengals and a six-time Pro Bowl selection. He is an Alzheimer's
Association Champion and has testified in Washington, D.C., for
increased funding for Alzheimer research.*

*I*t has become a ritual. Every game, no matter what's going on, no matter where I am
on the football field, I look around the stadium and my grandmother, Alice Black, will
instantly pop into my head. I see her clear as a bell.

That's understandable. I spent most of my life under my grandmother's roof, under her
supervision. She was my backbone. She was the love of my life.

I never saw the Alzheimer's coming. I had honestly felt I would have her around for years
to talk to, laugh with and watch her enjoying her great-grandchildren. It wasn't to be. In
1996, my rookie year in San Francisco, we got the diagnosis.

The disease took her mind away. She never really understood I was becoming a professional player and what that meant. She never understood that she didn't have to buy me
clothes anymore and put them on layaway. I don't even know if she understood that I owe
my life and success to her.

My grandmother helped mold me into the person I am today. She helped raise me, my
brother and sisters in her home, while my young mother was out working numerous jobs.
I wasn't the sweetest and nicest kid growing up, and I'm pretty sure I gave her a lot of
headaches.

It's true, she was extremely strict, but that's the way she was raised herself. She didn't
let us go out and play or run around on the street unsupervised. But she did the best she
could, and her parenting gave me many gifts.

My grandmother taught me the self-discipline, focus and work ethic that have powered
my success. If I'm strong-willed and strong-minded, it's because I learned that from her.
She taught me to be proud of who I am and to never back down or take a back seat to

anyone. I'm proud to be Alice Black's grandson. Anything I do for her today will never be enough to match what she did for me.

But it doesn't matter how much fame and privilege I've gained through football, how many hundreds of passes I catch, how many touchdowns I score. I can't do one thing myself to cure my grandmother or slow her disease down.

> 66 *The disease took her mind away. She never really understood I was becoming a professional player and what that meant.* 99

That's why I'm blessed to be part of the Alzheimer's Association, using my status and my voice to heighten public awareness and get increased funding for research. Together, we can make a difference and defeat this horrible disease once and for all.

Today my grandmother can't walk anymore and is confined to a wheelchair. Sometimes she gives you a look that makes you think she wants to say something and can't, but then a smile on her face says it all.

If someone in your family has just been diagnosed with Alzheimer's, all I can tell you is to enjoy the time you have with them today. If they can still recognize and talk to you, cherish those moments, because they won't last.

And also try to hold on to your memories of the wonderful times you've shared in the past. That's what I'm doing when my grandmother's image comes to me on the football field.

For Memory

By Terry Moran, co-anchor of ABC News' Nightline

*T*en years after her death, it is my mother's needlework that now calls me back to her prime, to her grace, and helps me hear once again the sound of her laughter.

She had a fine hand with a needle, as they used to say. Pillowcases and canvasses, wall hangings and purses, abstract, figurative, decorative—so much craft and loveliness spun from her fingers as she sat under the lamplight, her glasses perched on the end of her nose, her feet tucked under her on the sofa, as the conversation of her family—a husband of 36 years, 10 children—carried on around her. Or perhaps more often, the noise of whatever we were watching on TV came from the sturdy wooden console to fill the room. She loved old movies and Major League Baseball: "They're playing long ball with that pitcher. Time to pull him!"

Without missing a stitch, she'd join the conversation, offering an opinion or sometimes a line of poetry; the Brownings were favorites. And sometimes, the steady, intricate minuet of needle and thread would cease, and she'd drop her hands into her lap, throw her head back and laugh. My mother had a wonderful sense of humor—a rich, almost fatalistic appreciation of life's occasional absurdities. I miss her so much.

We hardly noticed it at first. She'd stop in her needlepoint, look at her work in surprise and say, "Where was I?" And then she'd count her way back into her place and carry on.

The interruptions grew more frequent. The counting became harder. And eventually all that was left in her lap, under the blank gaze of Alzheimer's, was a canvas ragged with confusion, streaming threads like spilled paint or weeds grown up to choke a rose garden. The minuet stumbled, slowed, ended.

What Alzheimer's takes from a person is so precious, so profound, it just plain breaks your heart. And yet it is in that loss, in that suffering, that we find our calling in this cause. And I believe we find a paradoxical gift as well.

We must defeat Alzheimer's. For all the families out there who face the sorrow of losing a loved one to this disease, for all those men and women who face the loss of self and talent and relationships—we must achieve a world without Alzheimer's. Each of us has work to do—to raise consciousness, support our caregivers, inspire our government to action.

> ❝ *What Alzheimer's takes from a person is so precious, so profound, it just plain breaks your heart.* ❞

As we do so, let us appreciate that we who have been touched by Alzheimer's are given a special witness, a special understanding of how deeply interdependent all of us—each and every one of us—are upon one another. And how precious are the days we have together.

I'm lucky. I have the work of my mother's hands, her needlepoint masterpieces, to take me back along the current of memory to her, and to that lamplight, and to the sound of her laughter.

For memory, then, and the love it holds, we will prevail.

Taking on Alzheimer's

How Is Our Nation Responding?

Chapter 7

Strategy to Combat Alzheimer's Disease

By former House Speaker Newt Gingrich and former Nebraska Senator Bob Kerrey, co-chairs of the Alzheimer's Study Group, which published A National Alzheimer's Strategic Plan: The Report of the Alzheimer's Study Group *in 2009.*

Alzheimer's disease is looming as a national crisis. To look for solutions, the bipartisan Alzheimer's Study Group (ASG) we chaired—including such notables as former Supreme Court Justice Sandra Day O'Connor, former Surgeon General Dr. David Satcher and Nobel Laureate Dr. Harold Varmus—was commissioned by Congress and the Alzheimer's Association.

The cost of Alzheimer's is staggering. The average annual cost of health and long-term care for people with Alzheimer's is $33,007 per year, more than three times the average cost of $10,603 incurred by individuals 65 and older without this condition. We projected that the cost to the U.S. government will be $20 trillion through 2050. Recent reports from the Alzheimer Association, Dartmouth University and the Lewin Group confirm these findings. But the enormous impact Alzheimer's disease will have on the federal budget doesn't even begin to compare to the devastating impact of the disease on the fabric of America's families.

In Alzheimer families, both the patient and caregiver are forever changed. The impact is especially felt by women. Women are more likely than men to have Alzheimer's disease and other dementias. More than 20 percent of women reaching age 65 ultimately develop dementia (estimated lifetime risk), compared with approximately 17 percent of men. For Alzheimer's, the estimated lifetime risk is nearly one in five for women, compared with one in ten for men.

Those numbers are especially alarming when we consider that most caregivers for people with Alzheimer's are women. We know many women don't perceive themselves as caregivers but simply as loving family members doing what they're supposed to do. This lack of self-acknowledgement doesn't alleviate the impact on the caregivers' own lives. Studies show that women who care for people with Alzheimer's are at increased risk for depression and anxiety and twice as likely as other women to develop cardiovascular disease. That's the toll taken by the daily physical, mental and emotional stress of having to dress, bathe, feed and medicate loved ones, deal with sometimes violent outbursts and constantly worry that their patients will hurt themselves or wander away.

And the burden on women is even heavier than that. Many of them in the so-called Sandwich Generation care not only for ill parents but for their own children as well. And so often this full-time caregiving job is on top of a full-time paying job out in the workplace. The superhuman workload and additional stress eat away not just at the health of these women but at their strength and resolve, too. So while Alzheimer's will take a big chunk out of the American budget, it's also taking a big chunk out of millions of women's lives.

So how can we combat Alzheimer's disease? *A National Alzheimer's Strategic Plan: The Report of the Alzheimer's Study Group* provided three essential solutions to the Alzheimer epidemic:

The Alzheimer's Prevention Initiative: As a national priority, urgently focus on developing research into therapies to delay and ultimately prevent Alzheimer's disease. This capability will depend on streamlining the pathway for medical researchers working on the disease.

The Alzheimer's Care Improvement Initiative: To upgrade the quality of care, by 2012, institute a system to use value-based payments to reimburse providers for at least 20 percent of health and social services for people with dementia, and for 50 percent of these services by 2016. Value-based payments will reward healthcare and social services professionals who provide the high-quality coordinated care people with dementia most need for better health and a higher quality of life.

The Alzheimer's Public-Private Partnership: By the end of 2010, establish an outcomes-oriented, project-focused Alzheimer's Solutions Project Office within the federal government to lead the successful implementation of the Alzheimer's Prevention and the Alzheimer's Care Improvement initiatives.

(The full report can be found at www.alz.org/documents/national/report_ASG_alzplan.pdf.)

Support of these three important initiatives is growing. Bipartisan legislation has been introduced in the U.S. House of Representatives, the U.S. Senate and in state legislatures. Caregivers are uniting behind the science, and now—finally—government is uniting to put caregivers into the equation and get them help. That means help for American women.

Above all, our ultimate goal is to prevent, slow or cure Alzheimer's disease. Let's keep our eye on the prize.

Increasing Our Investment

By Senator Susan M. Collins (R-Maine), co-chair of the Bipartisan Congressional Task Force on Alzheimer's, co-sponsor of the Alzheimer's Breakthrough Act and co-author of the National Alzheimer's Project Act

As someone whose family has experienced the pain of Alzheimer's many times, I know that there is no more helpless feeling than to watch the progression of this devastating disease. More than 5 million Americans have Alzheimer's disease—including about 30,000 people in my home state of Maine. This number has doubled since 1980 and is expected to reach up to 16 million by the year 2050, when an estimated 15 percent of Americans age 65 and older will have the condition. This disease takes a tremendous personal and economic toll on both the individual and the family.

Moreover, Alzheimer's currently costs the United States $172 billion a year, primarily in nursing home and other long-term care costs. This figure will increase exponentially as the baby boom generation ages and is expected to top $1 trillion a year by 2050, according to a recent report by the Alzheimer's Association.

As baby boomers move into the years of highest risk for Alzheimer's disease, a strong and sustained research effort is our best tool to slow the progression and prevent the onset of this disease. Our investments in Alzheimer's have begun to pay dividends. Effective treatments for Alzheimer's disease are tantalizingly within our grasp. Unfortunately, however, while the number of Alzheimer cases has continued to climb, funding has been flat over the past five years and research is underfunded. For every dollar the federal government spends today on the costs of Alzheimer care, it invests less than a penny in research to find a cure.

We must increase our investment in Alzheimer research. We have made tremendous progress, but this is no time to take our foot off the accelerator. That is why, as the Senate co-chair of the Bipartisan Congressional Task Force on Alzheimer's Disease, I am an original cosponsor of the Alzheimer's Breakthrough Act. This bipartisan legislation would increase the funding for Alzheimer research at the National Institutes of Health to $2 billion, demonstrating the level of commitment warranted to advance the treatment and ultimately prevention of this disease.

This legislation would also provide much needed support for people with Alzheimer's and their families by increasing funding for the National Family Caregiver Support Program and by providing a tax credit of up to $3,000 to help families meet the costs of caring for a loved one. In addition to the terrible personal toll of Alzheimer's, this disease can devastate a family economically. These families need and deserve our help.

Along with Senator Evan Bayh (D-Ind.), I have also authored bipartisan legislation, the National Alzheimer's Project Act, to create the country's first national office responsible for leading government efforts to treat and prevent Alzheimer's disease. The National Alzheimer's Project Office would coordinate and oversee federal research to develop a plan to combat the disease and to eventually develop a cure. Our nation needs a more effective, coordinated national strategy aimed at preventing, delaying and finding a cure for Alzheimer's, and this legislation represents a critical step toward that goal. This legislation follows through on a key recommendation from the Alzheimer's Study Group.

Together, we have come a long way, but we have farther to go. I will continue to work with my colleagues to implement a national strategy that will move us forward in our battle against Alzheimer's.

Federal Response:
2010 Legislation

By Kathleen Sebelius, U.S. Secretary of Health and Human Services, who also served as Governor of Kansas and Kansas Insurance Commissioner

Alzheimer's is a heartbreaking disease. Anyone who has a loved one with Alzheimer's knows how hard it is to watch a spouse, partner, sibling or parent change before your eyes.

Alzheimer's is also changing our nation's population. As we live longer—and as the enormous wave of baby boomers moves into its senior years—the number of Americans with Alzheimer's will escalate, and so will the number of caregivers.

The impact will be huge. Just in 2010, the projected healthcare spending for people with Alzheimer's and other dementias is $172 billion. Medicare and Medicaid spend the majority of those healthcare dollars. While we are working to find a cure, finding a treatment that could even just slow down the progression of Alzheimer's by a few years would result in profound improvements in the lives of millions of Americans and could significantly decrease healthcare spending by the government, as well as individual families.

The federal government has always played an important role in Alzheimer research and care. But as the disease becomes more common, we have an important new weapon in the fight to support people with Alzheimer's and their families and ultimately find a cure. That is the Affordable Care Act, the comprehensive healthcare reform legislation passed by Congress and signed by President Obama earlier this year.

The Affordable Care Act will boost Alzheimer research by establishing a Cures Acceleration Network (CAN)—a new program at the National Institutes of Health (NIH) that's specifically focused on finding cures for diseases like Alzheimer's, where we've yet to discover widely effective treatments or medications. That's on top of the $10.4 billion in additional funding for the NIH in the American Recovery and Reinvestment Act—the largest boost to biomedical research in our history.

The CAN program will build upon current research efforts, which have already advanced our understanding of this terrible disease. In just the past year, three new genes that appear to play a role in Alzheimer's have been discovered, and we're making great strides in imaging and other techniques aimed at the earliest possible diagnosis and faster testing of potential new treatments.

The 2010 Affordable Care Act will also help people with Alzheimer's receive better care by moving us toward a patient-centered healthcare system that will be better able to meet their needs. For example, it establishes a new Center for Medicare & Medicaid Innovation that will begin testing new ways of delivering care. The center will be able to look at innovative programs that provide comprehensive and coordinated care for Medicare patients identified has having cognitive impairment or difficulty performing the tasks of everyday life. Moving toward programs that provide comprehensive care plans to treat a patient's full range of needs could be very effective for Americans with Alzheimer's.

Thanks to the Affordable Care Act, Americans with Alzheimer's will also have access to new resources to help them stay in their homes or communities.

A new "Independence at Home" program will provide coordinated primary care services for Medicare beneficiaries with multiple, complex medical issues, such as those faced by people with Alzheimer's.

The Community First Choice Option allows states to offer home- and community-based services to disabled individuals through Medicaid, rather than institutional care in nursing homes. That will keep people with Alzheimer's in familiar surroundings, closer to their friends and loved ones.

Finally, the new law will also increase federal Medicaid payments for states providing home- and community-based services to patients who might otherwise be placed in nursing homes. This builds on existing investments by the Administration on Aging in programs that provide community-based supports and services for persons with Alzheimer's disease and their family caregivers.

For all these programs to work—and to keep up with demand as the number of people with Alzheimer's escalates—we'll need a work force trained to care for them, from geriatric specialists to home healthcare aides. The Affordable Care Act helps supply these health professionals by investing in our primary care work force and by ensuring that nursing homes train their nursing aides to care for patients with special needs due to Alzheimer's or other dementias.

The Affordable Care Act also recognizes that most caregivers are not professionals but rather family members and friends. Today, the task of providing long-term care to people with Alzheimer's often falls to their children, especially their daughters—many of them in the Sandwich Generation, caring not just for their aging relatives but also for their own kids. To help these caregivers, the Affordable Care Act provides funding to train family members to understand and better manage the challenges of taking care of their loved ones.

For families who do opt for professional care, the cost is often exorbitant. The Affordable Care Act helps these families, too, by creating a voluntary insurance program called CLASS. It will provide cash benefits to adults who become disabled, including those who develop significant disability due to Alzheimer's and other cognitive impairments. Too few Americans today have long-term care insurance. With CLASS, more Americans will have some protection against the high cost of long-term care services and support for themselves or their family members down the road.

Combined, these reforms will accelerate Alzheimer research, improve care for people with Alzheimer's and ease the mounting burden on family caregivers. As the number of Americans with Alzheimer's grows, we need to step up our efforts to treat, prevent and ultimately cure the disease.

We have a long way left to go, but the Affordable Care Act is a huge step in the right direction.

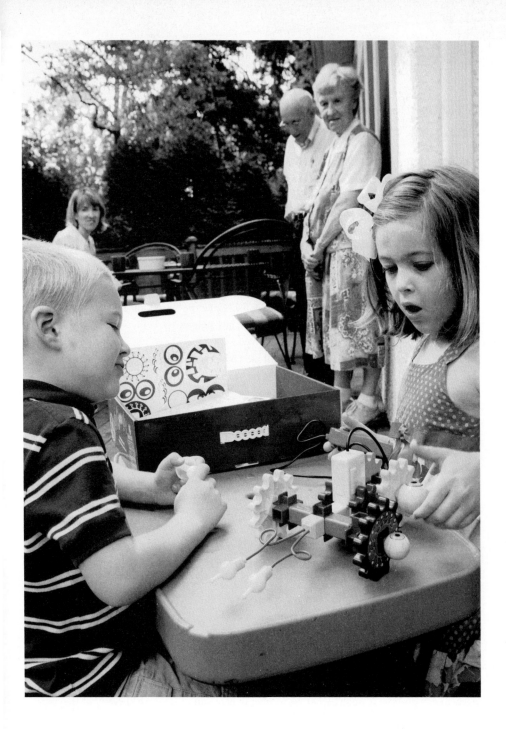

To Honor My Father

By Senator Barbara A. Mikulski (D-Md.), a member of the Bipartisan Congressional Task Force on Alzheimer's Disease who introduced the Alzheimer's Breakthrough Act to increase funding for Alzheimer research and the Family Assistance Act to create a tax credit for families caring for loved ones with chronic conditions like Alzheimer's

*W*hen you go to an Alzheimer's Association Memory Walk, which raises money for research and care, you hear people say, "I walk for Harry" or "I walk for Hillary"; "I walk for Josh" or "I walk for Juanita." Well, I walk for a guy named Mr. Willy.

Mr. Willy was my father: a quiet, wonderful man who owned a little grocery store in a blue-collar neighborhood in Baltimore. He had to leave school at a very young age, because he was from a large Polish family and everyone had to pitch in and support themselves. But he really understood the value of education, so he made sure my sisters and I had the best.

My father was committed to his community and family. He would often open the grocery store early, so local steelworkers could buy lunch before their morning shift. And Saturday nights, he would put records on and spend quality time at home, relaxing with my mother. He was so proud of all his girls.

And we were proud of him. We were so grateful for everything he gave us. He taught us important values: family, hard work, neighbor helping neighbor and heartfelt patriotism.

But as our father got older, his memory began to fail. The doctors would say, "Oh, it's just the stress of old age" or "It's just the depression of old age." He was misdiagnosed and given the wrong treatment. They prescribed tranquilizers and other medications to calm him down. Nothing helped, and he continued to go downhill.

But thanks to the Johns Hopkins Geriatric Center, we finally got the real diagnosis: Alzheimer's disease. It wasn't what we wanted to hear, but at least we knew what the problem was.

My father got sicker and sicker. He would have 36-hour periods when he couldn't tell day from night. He used language we had never heard him use before. As the disease progressed, it was devastating for him, heartbreaking for my mom and soul-wrenching for my sisters and me.

We felt powerless, and we were powerless. Though I was a United States Senator, though I could get the highest levels of the National Institutes of Health on the phone, though I could have a Nobel Prize winner from Johns Hopkins return my call, I could not help my father. No one knew how to slow or stop the course of this terrible disease.

My father would never have wanted a fancy tombstone to memorialize him. He would have said, "Barb, get out there and help the other guys. Get out there and work. And don't forget your mother." That's why I vowed to do everything I could—not just to support research, but also to create a safety net for Alzheimer families.

I know how difficult it is for the loved ones of the as many as 5.3 million Americans who have this disease. I know the toll that caring for a sick parent or spouse can take. That's why I have fought to increase funding for Alzheimer research, to establish a national summit on Alzheimer's and to make permanent a 24-hour call center for expert advice about Alzheimer treatment and resources. And I vow to continue to fight to support caregivers through tax credits, education and access to affordable, quality health care.

My father taught me that each of us can make a difference. Together we can make change happen. We must keep fighting until we find a cure for Alzheimer's.

State Government Gets Ready

Currently, 31 states have or are in the process of developing a State Alzheimer Plan. Here's a snapshot of what's happening in California:

California is at the leading edge of the coming Alzheimer epidemic. Right now, 10 percent of all people with Alzheimer's in the United States live in California.

That's why we're developing our own Alzheimer's Disease Plan, to be presented at the end of 2010 by our Alzheimer's Task Force—more than 30 policy leaders in health and aging, as well as family members and healthcare providers. They have received input from more than 2,500 family and professional caregivers, health and business leaders— gathered in community meetings, focus groups, and interviews and surveys conducted statewide in five languages.

In addition, much Alzheimer research is conducted in our state. For example, the California Institute for Regenerative Medicine has awarded five grants specifically for Alzheimer's disease stem cell therapy research. We continue to support our ten California Alzheimer's Disease Centers, training a critical healthcare work force in diagnostics and management of the disease. Our state has many other innovative programs including the Alzheimer's Disease and Related Disorders Research Fund, a state income tax check-off that has provided seed grants to new researchers and helped draw more federal research dollars to California. We're in the fight.

—California Governor Arnold Schwarzenegger

What One City Is Doing

Last year, our city's Alzheimer's/Dementia Expert Panel issued its report, *2020 Foresight: San Francisco's Strategy for Excellence in Dementia Care.* Our city has begun implementing its recommendations, which call for:

- low-cost initiatives for caregiver education and training, plus enhanced access to services

- a pilot project to improve care coordination

- promotion of guidelines and standards to ensure high-quality services

- policy initiatives to enable the better management of resources and an investment in community-based care that may reduce the use of more intensive, higher-cost services

- a demonstration project to create a chronic-care management system

Our goal is to improve the quality of life not only for San Franciscans with Alzheimer's but for their caregivers as well. For more information on *2020 Foresight: San Francisco's Strategy for Excellence in Dementia Care,* go to www.sfhsa.org/asset/ReportsDataResources/ 2020ForesightStrategyForExcellenceinDementiaCare.pdf

—San Francisco Mayor Gavin Newsom

Activating the Next Generation

By Alissa Anderegg,
a 16-year-old from Danville, California

My grandmother, Mary Fran Anderegg, has had Alzheimer's ever since I can remember. Over the years, it has hurt to watch the disease unfold.

It was so hard when I was younger when she would forget my name or ask me over and over again how old I was. She'd throw temper tantrums at the dinner table, scream at me, take my toys or bang on glass mirrors trying to figure out why her reflection wouldn't answer her. My grandma's behavior was sometimes so bad, it was as if she were the child, even though she was 70 years older than me. As a young girl, sometimes I wasn't sure if her behavior was her actual personality or if it was Alzheimer's that made her be mean to me and steal my Beanie Babies.

I could go on about the toll her Alzheimer's has taken on my family: the time and money spent taking care of her, the emotional stress we have all experienced or how in many ways I had to grow up fast at 8 years old when she came to live with us. But I like to have a positive attitude. Unfortunately, trying to stay positive about Alzheimer's can be a challenge for anyone, let alone kids who can't help thinking they're at fault for their grandparents' behavior.

There actually were positive moments. Even though she couldn't remember what she had for breakfast that morning, or anything that happened in the last 40 years for that matter, Grandma Mary Fran remembered a lot about her childhood and shared it with us. At dinner, she'd talk about her experiences growing up on her family's ranch in Texas. So whenever she'd act up, I used to imagine her being my age in a scene from *Little House on the Prairie*. I tried to remember that person, not the one who was screaming at me or sitting and staring blankly at the wall.

As I got older and Grandma Mary Fran's case progressed, I began to research more about the disease to better understand what she was going through. I learned that she wasn't really responsible for her actions, which were the result of Alzheimer's disease taking over her thought processes. She couldn't help it.

I eventually decided that I wanted to get involved in the cause. I started by giving reports about Alzheimer's in my middle school. In just one class, I was shocked when five other students raised their hands to say that they also had loved ones with Alzheimer's. That made me realize how children keep such experiences to themselves and don't reach out. I had also kept my struggles with my grandmother to myself, when I could have been getting support from adults and other children.

I knew that I could make a difference and reached out to volunteer in Alzheimer organizations. I created a Facebook group, Alz4Kidz & Alz4Teenz: Resources for Kids about Alzheimer's and was approached to be part of HBO's *The Alzheimer's Project.* This was also a learning experience for me.

The HBO producers asked me to interview Grandma Mary Fran's old friends to learn about her life before Alzheimer's. What a gift that was to me! I'm recommending to other kids that they interview their family members with Alzheimer's while they can.

When I did, I learned that she was such an amazing, accomplished woman, a leader and philanthropist in our community and state. Then when we took the camera crew to see my grandma, it was heartbreaking. This once-amazing woman now could no longer speak, eat or walk by herself. Alzheimer's had literally taken over.

At times I worry that other members of our family will develop Alzheimer's. All I can do is pray and spread my story. It is so important for teens to embrace the cause and use our voices to make a difference. By just spreading the word and sharing our experience, we honor our grandparents' lives and help other kids make sense of Alzheimer's.

Now is the time for us to come together to fight this disease that will affect more and more kids as time goes on.

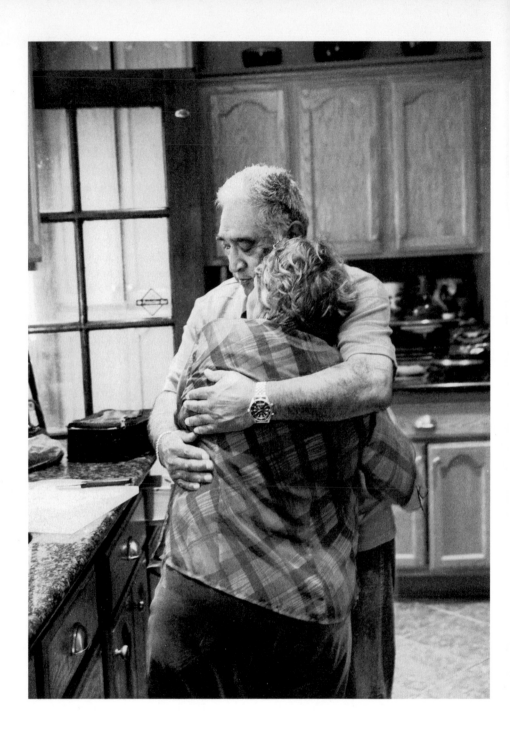

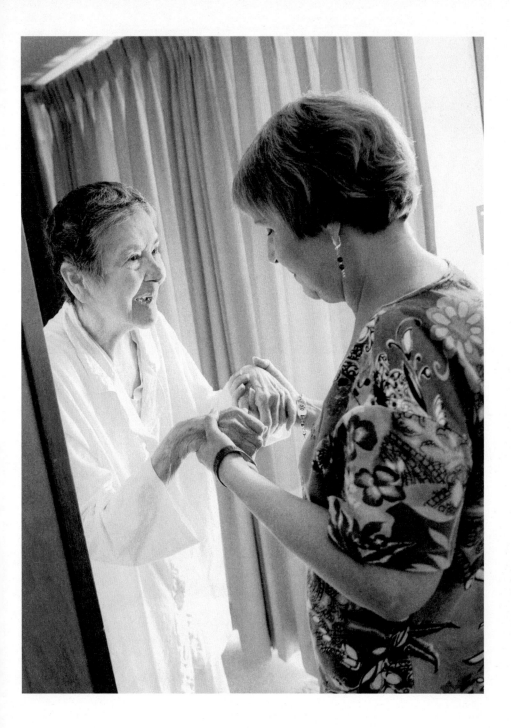

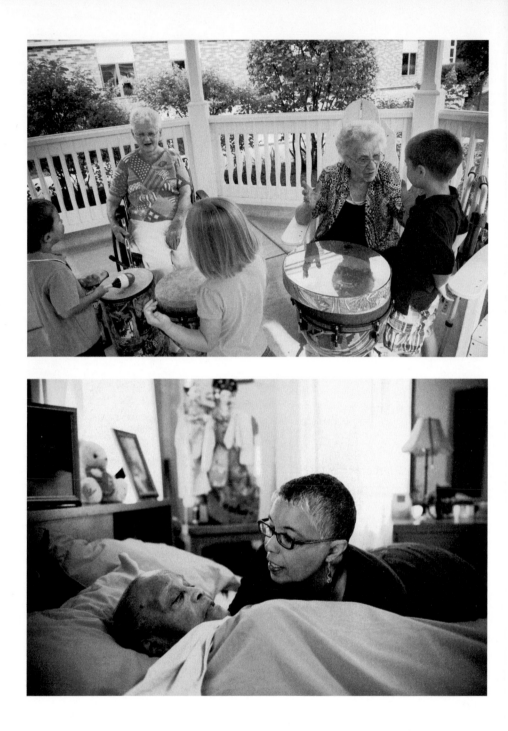

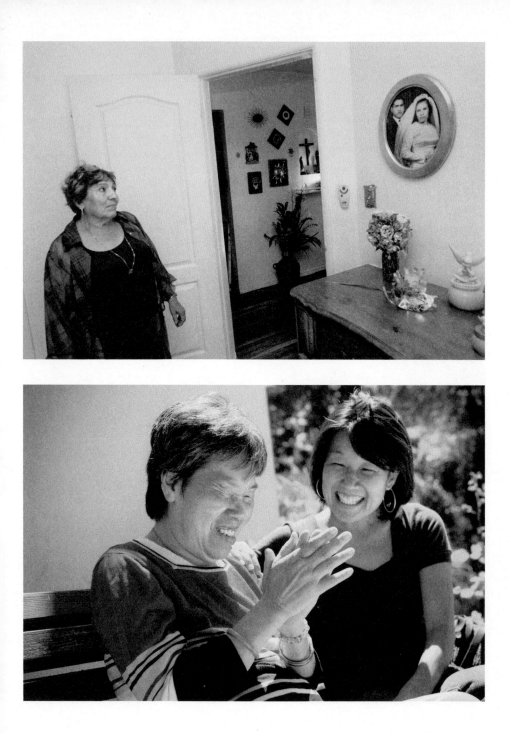

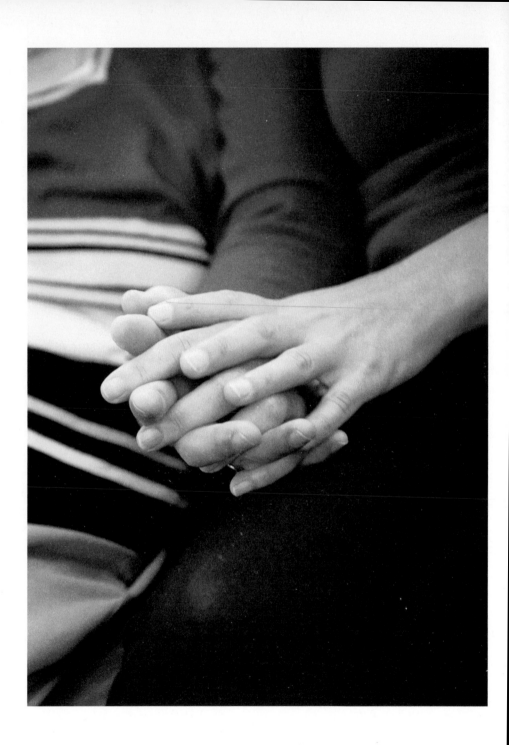

Conclusion

Why We Did This Report

By Harry Johns

My mother sat in her living room chair, in the same spot that had been hers for the nearly 50 years she had spent in her house. My brother sat in the companion chair to hers, the one my father had vacated almost 40 years earlier. I was on the couch, at the end closest to them. This was furniture that my brother and I were expected to respect in our younger years. On this day, my mother would consider neither of us respectful to her, even though that was far from true. Despite preparing with all of the best information on how to have the conversation, despite the fact that my brother and I were in agreement on the need for the discussion, and that we were following up on what my mother's doctor had already told her, our talk did not go smoothly. She acknowledged that she should not be driving, but she did not want to give up her keys.

One of 13 children born into Wabash River-bottom poverty during the Depression, my mother had been toughened by a challenging life. Widowed by a young husband while still young herself, she was abandoned with two young children by another. If not highly, formally educated, she had always been one of the sharpest people I've known. On the day we sat with her to talk about her no longer getting behind the wheel, she was much smaller than the 5'0" height she had always claimed. Her cognitive exams had shown greater impairment, and it was often quite apparent without the tests. Even so, she was still a strong presence. She wanted to preserve the option to drive "if necessary" in an "emergency." She also clearly sent the message that the two people she cared about most in the world had now abandoned her to side with her doctor. I don't recall ever having a more painful conversation.

Just as I had to come to grips with the matriarch of the family having Alzheimer's disease, so, too, have millions of other people. There are as many as 5.1 million Americans age 65 and older with Alzheimer's disease [1] and of them 3.3 million are women and 1.8 million are men.[2] Although this disease is devastating to all Americans, it is women—our mothers, grandmothers, sisters and aunts—who comprise almost 65 percent of those with the disease. Unless we discover effective treatments that prevent, delay the onset or progression, or cure Alzheimer's, in the next 40 years it will be our daughters who will make up the 8 million women with the disease by mid-century.[3]

Given my mom's Alzheimer's (she died three years ago) and my role as president and CEO of the Alzheimer's Association, I'm especially sensitive to the disproportionate effects of Alzheimer's on women demonstrated by *The Shriver Report on Women and Alzheimer's*. It's not difficult for me to understand why so many families are in denial about Alzheimer's. Facing it, like the disease itself, is terrible for everyone affected. Nonetheless, denial causes many with disease to go undiagnosed. It causes families to be completely unprepared for the realities that so many will face as it progresses, and we know anecdotally[4] that many physicians avoid diagnosing Alzheimer's because they don't want to be the bearer of such bad news. Some will simply prescribe available medications without making a diagnosis.

This anachronistic approach must change. We need to talk about Alzheimer's disease openly and widely until acceptance of its diagnosis and its discussion is commonplace. That's why Maria Shriver and her entire family speaking out about their father's condition is so vital. That's why the Alzheimer's Association is working with her on this very important report. That's why the Reagan family's discussion of President Reagan's Alzheimer diagnosis was so crucial in 1994, and why their work with the Alzheimer's Association has been so beneficial. It's also why the Alzheimer's Association has made it a high priority to raise the level of the discussion in America by annually releasing *Alzheimer's Disease Facts and Figures*; sponsoring the HBO series *The Alzheimer's Project*; working closely with the media to produce significantly increased coverage of Alzheimer's; placing advertising to create awareness; and working with other Champions like David Hyde Pierce, Kate Mulgrew, Victor Garber, Natalie Morales, Bradley Cooper, Soleil Moon Frye, Seth Rogen, Terrell Owens, Peter Gallagher and many others to get America talking about Alzheimer's.

We will know that we have reached yet another level of this vital public discussion when someone like a Hollywood celebrity or a sitting politician steps before the cameras early after diagnosis and unequivocally tells the world that he or she has Alzheimer's. This will be another turning point in the national discussion of this burgeoning epidemic.

One of the things I'm most proud of is the Alzheimer's Association's important role in providing individuals who have Alzheimer's disease with opportunities to speak out and tell the public directly what Alzheimer's does to their lives. One of the ways we do this is through our Early Stage Advisory Group. Our advisors help to inform our messages and

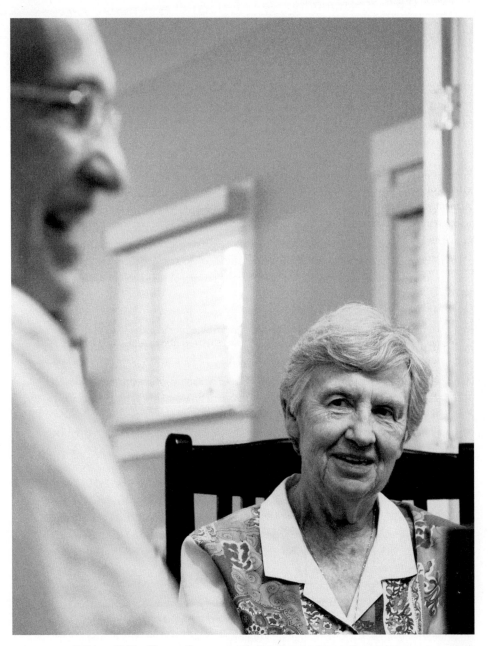
Kathleen Kahle, 77, was diagnosed with Alzheimer's disease five years ago.

provide valuable insight into what we do as we work alongside them to raise awareness and elevate concern. In fact, current and alumni members of our Early Stage Advisors, Kris Bakowski, Mary Ann Becklenberg and Mimi Steffens, have written essays contained in this report.

Because of so many remaining myths and misconceptions, it's important to say explicitly that Alzheimer's is not just a little memory loss. It's not normal aging. It's a progressive, degenerative and ultimately fatal disease. The problem is already so big that it is difficult to grasp the scale of the staggering numbers. With the aging of baby boomers like me, the current size of the epidemic—with its devastating impact on individuals with the disease, their caregivers and families, the medical system, our state and federal budgets and our economy—could be dwarfed by the growth of the problem during our lifetimes.

Right now, 5.3 million people are estimated to have Alzheimer's in the United States, including as many as 200,000 who are younger than 65.[5] If we don't successfully change the course of the disease, by the middle of the century as many as 16 million Americans could have Alzheimer's.[6] This overall incidence level doesn't capture the disproportionate effect on the women of America. One in six American women will have Alzheimer's during her lifetime. If she has a husband, one in ten of those men will ultimately have Alzheimer's,[7] creating the very real possibility that a woman will be a caregiver for her husband and then develop the disease herself.

As a result of such a high level of incidence, Alzheimer's is now the sixth-leading cause of death in the United States. The disease killed more than 74,000 individuals in 2007 (the last year with available statistics).[8] For perspective, that's more than breast cancer and prostate cancer combined. As reporting of diagnoses improves and the number of people with the disease is increased by the aging baby boomer population, deaths due to Alzheimer's will continue to rise.[9]

The economic factors of Alzheimer's rival the human devastation of the disease. According to the Alzheimer's Association's report *Changing the Trajectory of Alzheimer's Disease: A National Imperative*, we're spending $172 billion annually on Alzheimer's and other dementia care in America. $88 billion of that is for Medicare alone, which is 17 percent of the total Medicare budget.[10] Medicare beneficiaries with Alzheimer's or another dementia cost the system three times more than someone else 65 or older in Medicare who does not have a dementia.[11] For Medicaid, the cost multiplier for someone with dementia is nine times more than a comparable individual.[12]

The *Trajectory Report* also estimates that during the next 40 years, the cost of Alzheimer's and other dementias will exceed $20 trillion. Millions will get Alzheimer's and other dementias, and millions will suffer. Millions more will care for them and will suffer in different ways. So, it's going to cost us $20 trillion[13] and all we'll have to show for it is a long list of the dead, personal heartbreak and the devastating effects on caregivers and families.

Caregiving for Alzheimer's can literally take everything a caregiver has to give. The manifestation, the degeneration and the progression of the disease varies with the individual, but the broad outlines are the same. If diagnosed early, after symptoms have been recognized, the individual with the disease can enjoy a positive and functional (though impaired) life, sometimes even for a few years. However, the individual will eventually lose functions until caregivers must be available 24 hours a day, at home or in a residential care facility.

In one study of family caregivers, 59 percent of caregivers felt as though they were "on duty" 24 hours a day during the last year of life for the person with dementia.[14] 72 percent acknowledged that "they experienced relief when the person died."[15] A National Alliance for Caregiving and AARP study found that caregivers providing support for someone with Alzheimer's or another dementia were 31 percent more likely to reduce hours or quit work altogether when caring for someone without behavioral symptoms, when compared to caregivers of other older people.[16] For the similar group of individuals caring for someone with behavioral symptoms of Alzheimer's or another dementia, the comparative likelihood of needing to reduce hours or to quit a job was 68 percent.[17]

The Alzheimer's Association is the leading global voluntary health organization in Alzheimer care and support, and the largest nonprofit funder of Alzheimer research. Our mission is to eliminate Alzheimer's disease through the advancement of research; to provide and enhance care and support for all affected; and to reduce the risk of dementia through the promotion of brain health.

Our vision is a world without Alzheimer's, and since our founding in 1980, we have moved toward this goal by advancing research and providing support, information and education to those affected by Alzheimer's and related dementias. We provide information, care consultation at all stages of the disease, support groups and other community interventions to make a difference in the lives of those who have the disease and those who are affected by it.

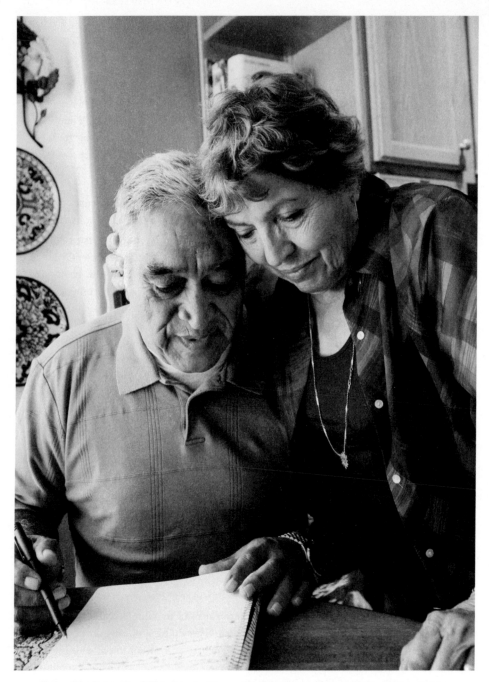

Before his diagnosis of Alzheimer's disease, Ricardo Flores often wrote love letters to his wife, Lidia. His handwriting may no longer be legible, but he still writes to her.

To find the ultimate answers to the disease, we fund cutting-edge research in top laboratories around the world. We support novel approaches that drive new thinking in the field. We fund science aimed at treatment and diagnosis as well as psychosocial interventions. And we annually convene the largest research meeting in the world, the Alzheimer's Association International Conference on Alzheimer's Disease (AAICAD), drawing together the global Alzheimer research community to advance the science.

The Alzheimer's Association is also the leading voice for Alzheimer's disease advocacy, fighting for critical Alzheimer research, prevention and care initiatives at the state and federal level. Among other important initiatives, we worked closely with the Social Security Administration on its inclusion of younger-onset Alzheimer's in their Compassionate Allowances Initiative to streamline approval of benefits for those diagnosed before age 65. And we worked with the U.S. Food and Drug Administration (FDA) to add people with dementia and their caregivers to FDA Advisory Panels as consultants.

In combination with our efforts, what's most needed in Alzheimer's is investment in more research to change the course of the disease as soon as possible. The science community is upbeat about the potential for Alzheimer advances, but as the boomer generation ages to the point of what is considered the earliest age of typical onset, 65, more dramatic increases in prevalence draw ever nearer. While one in eight of all of those over 65 have Alzheimer's, almost one in two of those over 85 have it.[18] We need to act. Now.

Based on the most recently available data, annual federal funding for cancer is about $6 billion, for cardiovascular disease about $4 billion and for HIV/AIDS about $3 billion. These are all important investments that should continue based on their high returns in lives saved.[19] Not counting the one-time stimulus funds, total federal funding for Alzheimer research is just $469 million.

Alzheimer's must be a national priority. I'm encouraged by the White House Briefing on the Challenge of Alzheimer's Disease in the United States in which I participated on World Alzheimer's Day, September 21, 2010. I believe it was a good step by this administration toward what we need: a real and sustained effort to change the course of Alzheimer's. But today, our federal government—in fact, our country as a whole—is not prepared for the worsening Alzheimer disaster.

We aren't funding enough research to stop it. We don't have a plan for handling the surging cost of care if it isn't stopped. We don't have enough residential care facilities for that inevitable point in the disease process when even the most dedicated caregivers can no longer handle the care at home. Do the math: Without even considering the human effects, Alzheimer's disease will cost our nation $1 trillion a year when a baby born in 2010 turns 40.[20] And, we're spending less than $500 million a year to avoid those costs. Should we invest more now to stop it, or wait and let that little baby pay the costs 40 years later? The answer is clear.

I get the benefit of exposure to scientists working worldwide to end this disease. I have the opportunity to see so many others dedicated to providing care and support to those who will have the disease before we finally cure it, and I see all of the volunteers, staff and donors who advance the mission of the Alzheimer's Association each and every day. Because of their collective energy, I remain optimistic about Alzheimer advances. I believe that we will succeed. We must. My mother lived a modest life, even after her sons could support her additional needs or wants, but she did always enjoy clothes. She was a seamstress for both vocation and avocation. She also always had shoes to go with those clothes. When my wife and brother and I were packing up and cleaning out the house she had lived in all those years, we discovered she owned a lot more shoes than we had previously realized! I have since joked that depending on your age group, you might compare her number of pairs to Imelda Marcos or Carrie Bradshaw.

As my brother and I worked in another room, my wife came in with one particular shoebox to show us. On the end of the box was a little note, in my mother's hand: "My Best Shoes." It hit me that at the moment of writing that note my mother must have realized her own future: she would soon be unable to recognize her own "best shoes." I was shaken because it was simultaneously so small and so simple a moment, yet so representative of what people with Alzheimer's face—and because no one should have to face it. No one—no mother, no sister, no father, no brother—should have to write such a note.

I'm confident that we will prevail against Alzheimer's. It's not a matter of "if," it's a matter of "when." But "when" needs to be sooner rather than later. It's too late for my mother and the millions more who have died or who have progressed too far in their disease. Until we realize our vision of a world without Alzheimer's, the Alzheimer's Association will keep pursuing every possible approach to support those facing the disease and to find the answers we need to end it.

ENDNOTES

1   Alzheimer's Association, *2010 Alzheimer's Disease Facts and Figures,* May 2010. Accessible at www
    .alz.org.

2   The 8 million figure was provided to the Alzheimer's Association by Denis Evans, M.D., on July 21,
    2010. Dr. Evans' research team calculated the number based on data published in the *Archives of Neu-
    rology.*

3   Ibid.

4   In addition to anecdotal knowledge, there are articles that suggest another reason—resistance of family
    members (Kirby, McGuire 1998). And general practitioners have rated the three most important reasons
    for withholding the diagnosis as the certainty of the diagnosis (153 GPs, 54 percent), the patient's wish
    to be told (113 GPs, 40 percent) and the patient's emotional stability (90 GPs, 32 percent) (Vasilass,
    Donaldson, 1998).

5   Alzheimer's Association, *2010 Alzheimer's Disease Facts and Figures,* May 2010.

6   Ibid.

7   Ibid.

8   J.Q. Xu, K.D. Kochanek, S.L. Murphy, B. Tejada-Vera, "Deaths: Final Data for 2007." *National vital statis-
    tics reports,* vol 58, no.19. Hyattsville, MD: National Center for Health Statistics; 2010.

9   Alzheimer's Association, *2010 Alzheimer's Disease Facts and Figures,* May 2010.

10 Alzheimer's Association, *Changing the Trajectory of Alzheimer's Disease: A National Imperative,* May
    2010.

11 Ibid.

12 Alzheimer's Association, *2010 Alzheimer's Disease Facts and Figures,* May 2010.

14 Ibid.

15 Ibid.

16 Ibid.

17 Ibid.

18 Ibid.

19 National Institutes of Health, Estimates of Funding for Various Research, Condition, and Disease Cat-
    egories (RCDC), 2010.

20 Alzheimer's Association, *Changing the Trajectory of Alzheimer's Disease: A National Imperative,* May
    2010.

Epilogue

By *Vice President Joseph R. Biden Jr.*

E very day, millions of families confront the emotional and financial challenges that come along with caring for a loved one with Alzheimer's, while those living with Alzheimer's worry about concerns that ultimately trouble us all—not becoming a burden, being with family, living with grace and dignity.

This report tells the full story of Alzheimer's in America by weaving compelling personal essays together with the latest information on medical research, caregiving and the economic impacts of the disease. It is largely a story of women caring for women, but it resonates with nearly every American. It is a story that raises many hard questions: How do we help a loved one live with this disease? How do we help our friends grapple with it? How do we make life easier for caregivers? How do we do more to improve treatment? There aren't easy answers to any of them. But one thing is clear: we must spare no effort in fighting this disease and supporting the families it has devastated.

I am optimistic that we are poised to make headway against Alzheimer's. The Obama administration has already invested hundreds of millions of dollars in Alzheimer research. In addition, the healthcare reform law signed by the president in March created a tax credit that will support small companies working on promising new therapies for diseases like Alzheimer's. It also established the "Cures Acceleration Network," a new program at the National Institutes of Health that will focus on speeding the development of cutting-edge treatments for devastating illnesses.

While we must make progress on treatment and diagnosis, we must also do more to support caregivers. Women, who are still much more likely to be the primary caregivers of people with Alzheimer's, now make up nearly half of the work force, and their earnings are indispensable in most American households. That's why supporting caregivers is not just a "women's issue"—it is a middle-class economic security issue, and it affects a staggering number of families. More than 40 percent of American workers have provided elder care for someone in the last five years, and most caregivers of people with Alzheimer's or other dementias work full or part-time.

Every caregiving situation is slightly different. To help respond to the needs of patients and to reduce the strain on families providing care, the Middle Class Task Force, which I chair, has proposed a new Caregiver Initiative. The initiative would provide additional funding for programs that provide temporary respite care, counseling and training for caregivers, transportation assistance and other services. Expanding access to flexible work arrangements has also been a priority of the task force and our entire administration—one that will become even more critical as the baby boomers age and an increasing number of Americans are juggling work and caregiving.

There is no more precious gift than caring for a loved one, but too often the cost of caregiving pushes families to the financial brink. That's why we have proposed a major expansion of the Child and Dependent Care Tax Credit, which can cover some of the costs associated with paying for the care of a spouse or parent with Alzheimer's. The Task Force will continue to examine policies aimed at addressing the financial consequences of caregiving.

Finally, as Secretary Sebelius discusses in her essay, the passage of comprehensive health reform was an important step forward. The new health reform law will improve the quality of care for people with Alzheimer's by creating training opportunities for both health professionals and family caregivers and by investing in research on new treatments and better ways to deliver care. It will promote early detection by requiring new insurance plans, as well as Medicare and Medicaid, to cover preventive services without charging deductibles or copayments.

The new law will also ease the strain on family budgets by reducing out-of pocket prescription drug costs for Medicare beneficiaries. And it creates a voluntary insurance program for long-term care services, which will help people with Alzheimer's remain independent for as long as possible.

Alzheimer's does not discriminate; sadly, it is a problem that touches almost everyone in America, regardless of race or class or political affiliation, at some point in their lives. It causes untold pain. The strength and resilience shown by people with Alzheimer's and their families is an inspiration, but that does not diminish their heartbreak.

Until we have cured this disease, there will always be plenty of work left to do. This report leaves no doubt that the challenges are immense. But countless scientists, doctors, advocates, policymakers and caregivers are wholly committed to making progress. There is hope—and we must not rest until Alzheimer's has ravaged its last mind.

Allies

A poem by Keven Bellows

Stay by my side, I silently command.
His familiar contours: my only safety,
his trusted hands: my touchstone
to a past where we never lost touch.
Though we still breath the same air
lay awake in the same big bed,
only I preserve the stores of our story.
His distant smile chills me.
Still, I must disarm my heart,
shield him with my body—
the one he brought to life long ago
and showed me how to wear.

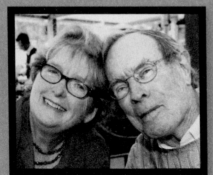

Keven Bellows and her husband Jim Bellows, who she lost to Alzheimer's disease in 2009.

"Allies" is from The Blue Darter (*Conflux Press*), a book of poems by Keven Bellows.

Appendix

Polling Methodology: Alzheimer's Association 2010 Women and Alzheimer's Poll

The Alzheimer's Association, in collaboration with *The Shriver Report on Women and Alzheimer's*, contacted 3,118 adults nationwide by telephone from August 25 to September 3, 2010. Telephone numbers were chosen randomly in separate samples of landline and cell-phone exchanges across the nation, allowing listed and unlisted numbers to be contacted, and multiple attempts were made to contact each number. Within households, individuals were randomly selected, and interviews were conducted in English and Spanish.

The survey includes "oversamples" of African-Americans and Hispanics, selected from census tracts with higher than 8 percent concentration of each respective group. It also includes an oversample of Asian-Americans using a listed sample of Asian-American households. The combined samples include: 2,295 white, non-Hispanic; 326 African-American; 309 Hispanic; 305 Asian; and 135 respondents of another race. These cases were weighted to account for differential probabilities of selection and to account for overlap in the landline and cell-phone sampling frames. The sample was adjusted to match census demographic benchmarks for gender, age, education, race/ethnicity, region and telephone service.

The resulting interviews (including the oversamples) comprise a probability-based, nationally representative sample of U.S. adults. The margin of sampling error is plus or minus approximately 2 percentage points at the 95 percent confidence interval. The margin of error for African-American subgroup estimates is 5 points and for Hispanic estimates is 6 points at the 95 percent confidence interval. For smaller subgroups, the margin of error may be higher.

The national survey includes 202 caregivers to persons with Alzheimer's or dementia. This was supplemented with 300 interviews from a listed sample of caregivers to people with Alzheimer's for a total of 502 caregiver interviews. A caregiver is defined as an adult over age 18 who, in the past 12 months, has provided unpaid care to a relative or friend age 50 or older who suffered from Alzheimer's or dementia. Unpaid care may include help with personal needs or household chores. It might be managing a person's finances, arranging for outside services or visiting regularly to see how they are doing.

The care recipient need not live with the caregiver. Unfortunately, there are no official demographic benchmarks for the Alzheimer caregiver population. As a substitute, we derived benchmark estimates for this population from the characteristics of the caregivers reached in the base survey, which are probability-based and nationally representative. The weight for the caregiver sample adjusts all 502 caregiver cases to the weighted estimates for gender and race/ethnicity derived from base survey of caregivers. This weighting adjusted for the fact that the caregivers reached through the listed sample were somewhat more likely to be female and white, non-Hispanic as compared to those reached in the probability-based component of the study. The caregiver sample is a stand-alone, non-probability sample and, therefore, the margin of error is not computed.

Questionnaire design and interviewing was conducted by Abt SRBI of New York. Susan Pinkus of S.H. Pinkus Research and Associates coordinated the polling and helped in the analysis of the poll.

Acknowledgments

Maria Shriver

With a wide-ranging and complex report such as this, there are a lot of people to thank—a lot of people who believed in the project and worked around the clock to make it happen.

First things first. There would be no project without Karen Skelton. Last year, she made *The Shriver Report: A Woman's Nation Changes Everything* come to life, and she has worked her brilliance yet again. Karen put the team together and kept it together and moving forward, until the mission was done. It's an honor to work with her. In so many areas of my life, I trust and rely on her wisdom, her political skills and her strategic vision. She is the can-do power behind these important reports, which I believe are helping shape our nation's discussion about women working and women growing old.

Olivia Morgan's brilliance is seen in every aspect of the report. She has been a critical adviser to me over the last two years and contributed greatly to how we have identified, described and illustrated transformational moments in American culture. She managed academic writers, elected officials and our diverse Advisory Council with grace, diplomacy and tough love, when necessary. She represents the best of our thinking, working, mothering and inspiring woman's nation. I hope we continue to work together for years to come.

I once again salute Rebecca Beland for her stamina, smarts and savvy, and she has been assisted at every step by the diligent work and brains of our teammate, Jordan Burke. I thank Roberta Hollander, my mentor in work and in life, who nurtured and edited the personal essays. She put together the most impressive collection of firsthand accounts about Alzheimer's ever gathered in one place, and she kept our team laughing and joyful throughout. Finally, thank you Angela Geiger and especially Kate Meyer of the Alzheimer's Association for inviting me to partner with them on this report. I believe in your mission to find a cure and to help the families of those living with the disease. I'm honored to be in this fight with you.

To all those who wrote personal essays and shared your journeys with us: I applaud your bravery, your honesty and your generosity. I truly believe you are helping others dealing with this terrible disease. Barbara Kinney's photographs have made these stories come to life, and I thank her for her talent and sensitivity. Thanks to editor Dale Fetherling for his steadiness, his wisdom and his ability to always go a step further than asked. I thank the brilliant writers of the main chapters of this report for pulling together all the strands of research and current thinking and then presenting them in a way we can all absorb and digest. The extraordinary pollster Susan Pinkus stepped in to help manage and execute our enormous public opinion survey, and her vast surveying expertise is always invaluable. Thanks to Matt Rallens for making our cover and design a work of art and to Kristina Schake and Marissa Moss for their continued belief that what we are saying matters enough to be pitched far and wide. And to my dear friend, Annie Liebovitz, for allowing me to use her picture of my dad with my brothers and me. My gratitude also goes out to Erin Stein and the incredible team at the Women's Conference and the First Lady's Office, who have helped with everything I do.

I'm also thankful to the members of our Advisory Committee and to our corporate partners—Deloitte, Visa, Ann O'Leary and the UC Berkeley Center on Health, Economic and Family Security, and Ellen Galinsky's Families and Work Institute—who stood behind this project. Thank you again to John Podesta and his wonderful team at the Center for American Progress for his continued support of our work to shine a light on women in America today. Along with our media partners, ABC News and *Time*, and our grassroots outreach partner AARP, we are able to spark a conversation that needs to be heard and debated around this nation and the world.

And finally to my family, especially my four brothers: Thank you all for allowing me to share our journey with this disease in such a public way. Thank you for trusting me, supporting me and believing that by talking about our journey, we can help others who have found themselves on the same road.

Most of all, to my parents, Eunice and Sargent Shriver: I love you both until the end of God's time.

Harry Johns

The Alzheimer's Association produces significant data about Alzheimer's disease facts, attitudes and issues. These data provide both a context and evidence base to media, public officials and the general public for the need to address Alzheimer's disease—the public health crisis of this generation.

The Alzheimer's Association also spends a lot of time listening. We listen to people with Alzheimer's disease, caregivers, families, researchers and collaborators and to our more than 500,000 volunteers. These stories and viewpoints inspire us to go further faster to provide better care and an ultimate cure.

This listening and data began to lead us in a new direction. We realized more and more that we were hearing from, and about, women. The concept of a women and Alzheimer's report is the strategic vision of Angela Geiger, chief strategy officer for the Alzheimer's Association. With her foresight, we decided to create a report, merging our dual strengths, people and science, to shine a bright light on the unique issues of women and Alzheimer's. We would create a report using data and personal stories to show the crushing impact of Alzheimer's on women and to demonstrate a path toward a different future. It is with sincere appreciation that I recognize Angela for her ability to make innovative projects and partnerships like this come to life.

In the very early stages, our first call was to Maria Shriver, Alzheimer advocate, and her incredible team, our collaborators on HBO's *The Alzheimer's Project*. We asked her to simply write the forward. Maria, being Maria, didn't stop there. She suggested we use the full power of A Women's Nation to shine not just a light but a million megawatt spotlight on this issue by focusing the second *The Shriver Report* on women and Alzheimer's. How could we refuse?

Not only did this result in the brainpower and enthusiasm of Maria Shriver, but also the sharp intellect, deep connections and amazing dedication of her Women's Nation team. So, our first thanks go to Maria for her leadership and all of her dedicated work. Then, to her great team: Karen Skelton and Olivia Morgan as well as Roberta Hollander, Rebecca Beland, Jordan Burke and Julia Wright. Erin Mulcahy Stein has been a great partner across all of our collaborations.

We're thrilled to work with old friends and Alzheimer's Association board members, volunteers, advocates and Champions, including Kris Bakowski, Mary Ann Becklenberg, Dr. Laurel Coleman, Meryl Comer, Eugene Fields, Phyllis George and family, Laura

Jones, Lindsey Jordan, Princess Yasmin Aga Khan, Kathy Mattea, Chris Matthews, Terry Moran, Terrell Owens, Xuan Quach and family and Mimi Steffen. Thanks to each of them and all of the essay authors for sharing their stories and perspectives. Thank you to the chapter authors and editor Dale Fetherling for working with new data on such tight deadlines. Photographer Barbara Kinney demonstrated a great compassion for the families photographed for this book, and it shines through. To the families and facilities that opened their lives and doors to ensure that we were able to capture the true impact of women and Alzheimer's, you have our sincere admiration and gratitude. We deeply appreciate the contributions of Vice President Joe Biden and HHS Secretary Kathleen Sebelius to this report, and we look forward to working with them to make Alzheimer solutions a national priority.

We know the media power of *Time* and ABC will extend the number of women exposed to this opportunity in exciting ways, both educating women about the facts and resources available but also to inspire them to get involved with the Alzheimer's Association to move this cause forward.

And this report wouldn't have been possible without the great work of Alzheimer's Association staff and support of the Alzheimer's Association leadership. My sincere appreciation goes to Kate Meyer, who has tackled this complex, challenging project with grace, smarts and a sense of humor. She led a team of dozens, and special thanks go to Matthew Baumgart, Katie Buffone, Maria Carrillo, Robert Egge, Sam Fazio, Erin Heintz, Niles Frantz, Leslie Fried, Matt Hickey, Mike Kobus, Mary Beth Lantzy, Katie Maslow, Cynthia Strohschein, Bill Thies, Toni Williams and Marykate Wilson.

Finally, we thank all the women who are already part of the movement to change the course of Alzheimer's disease: mothers, grandmothers, sisters, aunts, partners, wives, daughters and friends who've been, or will be, touched by Alzheimer's. We will fight with you, and for you, for better care, better treatments and a cure.

About the Contributors

Maria Shriver is the author of six books and an Emmy- and Peabody Award-winning broadcast journalist currently serving as First Lady of California. Shriver was co-executive producer of last year's Emmy Award-winning four-part HBO documentary series, *The Alzheimer's Project,* which took an inside look at cutting-edge research in the country's leading Alzheimer laboratories and examined the effects of Alzheimer's on people with the disease and their families. One of the series' films, *Grandpa, Do You Know Who I Am?* was based on Shriver's best-selling children's book dealing with Alzheimer's.

A mother of four, Shriver has expanded the California Women's Conference into a star-studded, multi-day event for 30,000 participants, featuring newsmakers, cultural leaders and opinion makers, all with the goal of inspiring and empowering women to be Architects of Change in their own lives, their communities and the world.

Harry Johns became the president and chief executive officer of the Alzheimer's Association in September 2005. Since his arrival, the Association has launched new initiatives to advance the Alzheimer cause, including the first nationwide campaign to increase understanding and awareness about Alzheimer's; a project to accelerate treatment progress by promoting participation in clinical studies; and a variety of program offerings designed to support both individuals with the disease and their caregivers. He has substantially increased both revenue and program expenditures to support the mission of the organization.

Prior to joining the Alzheimer's Association, Johns spent more than 22 years in various positions with the American Cancer Society (ACS). In his final role at ACS, he served as the executive vice president for strategic initiatives and as a member of the four-person executive team. He was responsible for nationwide strategy, including information delivery, community programs, advocacy, marketing and fundraising. Johns earned a bachelor's degree in business administration from Eckerd College in St. Petersburg, Florida, and a master's degree in business administration from the Kellogg Graduate School of Management at Northwestern University in Evanston, Illinois.

Karen Skelton is the chief executive officer for *The Shriver Report*, a multi-year project updating the modern portrait of the American woman by examining transformational moments in American culture and society. She has been an advisor, strategist, campaign manager and field organizer on some of the most complex, groundbreaking and entrepreneurial projects in the nation. Skelton founded the California office of the Dewey Square Group and grew the multimillion-dollar California consulting practice from the ground up.

Since 2003, Skelton has worked as the executive co-producer and program director for the California Governor and First Lady's Women's Conference. Under the direction of Maria Shriver, she manages all aspects of programming for the world's premier live event for women, including helping to manage its growth and success, as well as preparing, scripting and designing authentic and meaningful conversations for over 500 world-famous newsmakers and private citizens. Skelton previously worked in the White House during the Clinton administration on the political staff and as a member of the defense team that argued against the impeachment of the president. Skelton served as the first director of political affairs for then-Vice President Al Gore, initiating and managing his first national political program in preparation for his 2000 election campaign. Skelton is a working mom who lives with her husband and daughters in Sacramento, California.

Angela Timashenka Geiger is chief strategy officer of the Alzheimer's Association, where she coordinates efforts to maximize the Association's strategic impact. Geiger also leads the Constituent Relations team to develop and deliver marketing, mass market fundraising and programmatic offerings to improve the Association's effects on the disease. Prior to joining the Alzheimer's Association, Geiger spent eight years at the American Cancer Society in a variety of customer-focused leadership roles in the areas of mission delivery, fundraising and marketing. She has her BA and MBA from the University of Pittsburgh.

Olivia Morgan is the former executive director of the Children's Health Forum and a former principal of the Dewey Square Group, where she worked on communications strategies with a special emphasis on nonprofit development. She served as the director of federal relations for California Governor Gray Davis and as a spokesperson for elected leaders at national and state levels. In addition to serving on the board of the Children's Health Forum, Morgan serves on the advisory board of the New England Center for Children and is honored to be a member of the President's Committee on the Arts and the Humanities. She is managing editor of *The Shriver Report*.

Kathryn (Kate) Meyer joined the Alzheimer's Association in 2004 and is a senior associate director of public relations. Meyer manages many of the national media and communications efforts to raise critically needed awareness about Alzheimer's disease and the Association. She also works closely with Association celebrity Champions dedicated to activating people to take action in the fight against Alzheimer's. Prior to joining the Alzheimer's Association, Meyer spent four years at Edelman Public Relations in Chicago with the corporate reputation management division and two years as a member of the Big Ten Conference media relations team. She has her BA from Purdue University.

Roberta Hollander is an award-winning writer and producer who worked at CBS News for 35 years, starting at CBS Radio, where she wrote hourly newscasts and commentaries for the likes of Douglas Edwards and Walter Cronkite. She moved on to television and the *CBS Morning News,* producing pieces for correspondents Hughes Rudd, Charles Kuralt and Maria Shriver, among many others. Hollander went on to work on the *CBS Evening News* through this year, also contributing to *CBS News Sunday Morning.* She has traveled the country and overseas, covering everything from political campaigns and conventions to earthquakes, floods and fires, Mars missions and Hollywood. Though she has won Emmys and a Peabody, her proudest achievement is her award from the Writers Guild of America.

Barbara Kinney is an award-winning photojournalist whose work has appeared on the covers of *Time, Newsweek* and *People* magazines. She was a White House photographer during the Clinton administration and was Hillary Clinton's campaign photographer during the 2008 presidential primary elections. She has traveled internationally, photographing projects for the Bill & Melinda Gates Foundation, the Clinton Foundation, CARE and the Eastern Congo Initiative. Kinney has previously been a staff photo editor at *USA Today,* Reuters News Pictures and *The Seattle Times* and is a graduate of the William Allen White School of Journalism at the University of Kansas. To view more of her photography, visit www.barbarakinney.com.

Rebecca Beland is a Sacramento, California, native and a senior associate at the Dewey Square Group. She currently serves as the deputy director for *The Shriver Report* and the development associate for the California Governor and First Lady's Conference on Women. Beland has worked on a variety of high-profile projects, including last year's *The Shriver Report: A Woman's Nation Changes Everything.* She is a graduate of New York University and lives in San Francisco.

Matt Hickey has worked in a number of editorial capacities with the Alzheimer's Association since 2001, including serving as the editor of Insite, the Association's intranet, since 2003. A 1987 graduate of Ohio University with a bachelor's degree in journalism, he is a nationally published freelance writer on diverse subjects such as Major League Baseball, indie rock and foodservice management.

Cynthia Strohschein joined the Alzheimer's Association in 2003 and is the senior associate director of constituent marketing. Strohschein manages production of key publications and videos for the Association and oversees execution of marketing strategy for the Association's national and international conferences. Before joining the Alzheimer's Association, Strohschein worked as director of communications at Lakefront Supportive Housing. She is a former award-winning reporter for several newspapers throughout the Chicago suburbs and has her bachelor's degree from Loras College.

Jordan Burke is an associate at Plouffe Strategies and a native of Cape Elizabeth, Maine. His work on numerous national projects is focused on political and non-political communication, research and digital strategy. Burke held leadership positions in various states during the Obama presidential campaign. He lives in Washington, D.C.

Kelly Daley is a senior analyst at Abt SRBI, where she specializes in survey questionnaire design and data analysis across a variety of subject matters including public health, civic engagement and women's studies. Prior to joining Abt SRBI, she was co-director of the University of Chicago Survey Lab. Daley holds a Ph.D. in sociology from the University of Chicago and a masters degree in policy studies from The Johns Hopkins University.

Lisa Bain is a science and medical writer with a special interest in Alzheimer's disease and other neurodegenerative diseases. Over her 25-year career, she has authored three books and published widely in both the scholarly and lay literature.

Chapter Contributors

Maria C. Carrillo, Ph.D., is director of medical and scientific relations of the Alzheimer's Association. Dr. Carrillo oversees the Association's granting process and communication of scientific findings within and outside of the organization and is responsible for guiding the Scientific Grant Program, the mechanism through which the Association funds research applications. In addition to ensuring the smooth review of applications and distribution of awards to successful applicants, she is responsible for sharing results and ongoing investigations with a wide range of constituents.

Dr. Carrillo is a member of the Genworth Financial Medical Advisory Board. She received her Ph.D. from Northwestern University's Institute for Neuroscience in 1996. Since graduating from Northwestern, she completed a postdoctoral fellowship in the Neurology Department at Rush-Presbyterian-St. Luke's Medical Center in Chicago, where she was later hired as an assistant professor in the department of Neurological Sciences.

Bethany Coston is a Ph.D. candidate at Stony Brook University. She has published numerous book reviews and presented at conferences for her work on men, sexuality and violence. She is currently pursuing a dissertation on intimate partner violence in GLBTQ relationships, in the hopes that her efforts will open a dialogue about the social health crisis that very few currently acknowledge.

Sam Fazio, Ph.D., is director of special projects with the Alzheimer's Association. Dr. Fazio has worked for the national headquarters of the Alzheimer's Association since 1994 in a variety of areas, including education and training and program services. He currently works in the Medical and Scientific Relations area, where he oversees the international research conferences, scientific journal and social/behavioral research initiatives. Dr. Fazio also is involved in several research projects with older adults in the Chicago area related to the persistence of self, person-centered care, and health and wellness. Additionally, Dr. Fazio is a part-time faculty member in the gerontology program at Northeastern Illinois University in Chicago.

Dr. Fazio received his doctorate in developmental psychology from Loyola University Chicago. Prior to working for the Alzheimer's Association, Dr. Fazio worked for Rush-Presbyterian-St. Luke's Medical Center at the Alzheimer's Family Care Center, an adult day center specifically designed for people with dementia. He has worked in the field of aging since 1987 and has a broad range of experience, including research, leadership and management, working with older adults, families and direct care. Dr. Fazio is the author of *The Enduring Self in People with Alzheimer's: Getting to the Heart of Individualized Care* and co-author of *Rethinking Alzheimer's Care*.

Dale Fetherling, a journalist, author and teacher, has written or co-authored 16 books, varying from biographies to self-help to history. He holds a master's degree in journalism from Northwestern University and was a reporter and editor for major metropolitan newspapers, including *The Minneapolis Tribune* and *The Los Angeles Times*. For 15 years he was the editor of *The Los Angeles Times'* San Diego County Edition. He has taught reporting, writing and editing at six colleges and universities and speaks/presents at writing conferences and workshops.

Brent Fulton, Ph.D., is an assistant research economist at the Nicholas C. Petris Center on Health Care Markets and Consumer Welfare in the School of Public Health at University of California, Berkeley. Fulton received his doctorate in public policy analysis from the Pardee RAND Graduate School, where he focused on microeconomics and econometrics. His current research includes health economic topics, such as healthcare insurance and financing reform, pay for performance, health work force needs and attention-deficit/hyperactivity disorder. Brent received his MBA from UCLA and his BS from the U.S. Air Force Academy.

Michael Kimmel is professor of sociology at Stony Brook University He is the author of many books on contemporary masculinity, including *Manhood in America* and *Guyland*.

Katie Maslow is a consultant on Alzheimer's, dementia and aging issues. From 1995 to June 2010, she worked for the Alzheimer's Association, focusing on policy and practice initiatives to improve the quality, coordination and outcomes of health care and long-term care services and supports for people with Alzheimer's and other dementias and to increase support for family caregivers. Prior to joining the Alzheimer's Association in 1995, she was a policy analyst and senior associate at the U.S. Office of Technology Assessment (OTA), a congressional research agency. She has a bachelor's degree in sociology and psychology from Stanford University and a master's degree in social work from Howard University.

Ann O'Leary is executive director of the Berkeley Center on Health, Economic & Family Security (Berkeley CHEFS) at the University of California, Berkeley, School of Law and a senior fellow with the Center for American Progress. Previously, O'Leary served as a deputy city attorney for the city of San Francisco, a law clerk to U.S. Ninth Circuit Court of Appeals Judge John T. Noonan Jr. and from 2001 to 2003 as legislative director for senator Hillary Rodham Clinton (D-N.Y.). Prior to that, O'Leary served in a number of positions in the Clinton administration, including as special assistant to the president in the Domestic Policy Council, policy advisor to the First Lady and senior policy advisor to the Secretary of Education. She sits on the boards of Public Advocates and the East Bay Community Law Center.

O'Leary also served as a volunteer policy advisor to the Hillary Clinton for President campaign on issues related to children and working families and on the Obama-Biden Transition Team, where she advised the incoming administration on early childhood education issues. Together with Heather Boushey, O'Leary co-edited *The Shriver Report: A Woman's Nation Changes Everything.* O'Leary received her bachelor's degree from Mount Holyoke College, her master's degree from Stanford University and her law degree from University of California, Berkeley, School of Law.

John Podesta is president and CEO of the Center for American Progress. Under his leadership, the center has become a notable leader in the development of and advocacy for progressive policy. Prior to founding the center in 2003, Podesta served as White House Chief of Staff to President William J. Clinton. Most recently, Podesta served as co-chair of President Barack Obama's transition. Additionally, Podesta has held numerous positions on Capitol Hill. Podesta is a graduate of Knox College and the Georgetown University Law Center, where he is currently a visiting professor of law. He also authored *The Power of Progress: How America's Progressives Can (Once Again) Save Our Economy, Our Climate and Our Country.*